Natural Healing
Self Empowerment

The Ultimate Self Help Health Guide

By

The Polytope Press Research Group

Polytope Press
PO Box 1349
Phoenix AZ 85001

Natural Healing Self Empowerment

Copyright© 2004 by Polytope Press.
PO Box 1349
Phoenix AZ 85001
ISBN 0-9670526-6-1

First Printing
Printed in the USA

Thoreau Quotes

"It is the luxurious and the dissipated who set the fashions which the herd so diligently follow."

"Shams and delusions are esteemed for the soundest truths, while reality is fabulous."

"The universe is wider than our views of it."

"The minority is powerless while it conforms to the majority."

"From the hearth to the field is a great distance."

"I cannot spare my moonlight and my mountains for the best of man I am likely to get in exchange."

"They wanted me to agree not to breathe in the neighborhood of their paper castles. If I should draw a long breath, their weak and flabby sides would fall out… for my own inspiration would exhaust the air about them."

"There are a thousand hacking at the branches of evil to one who is striking at the root."

"Age is no better, hardly so well, qualified for an instructor as youth, for it has not profited so much as it has lost."

"What old people say you cannot do, you try and find that you can."

"There are as many ways as there can be drawn radii from one center."

"Rather than love, than money, than fame, give me truth."

"How to make the getting of our living poetic—for if it is not poetic, it is not life but death that we get."

"A man sits as many risks as he runs."

"For an impenetrable shield, stand inside yourself."

"Every man is the builder of a temple called his body to the god he worships after a style purely his own."

"Know your own bone. Do what you love. Gnaw it, bury it, unearth it, and gnaw it still."

"All that a man has to say or do that could possibly concern mankind is in some shape or other to tell the story of his love—to sing—and if he is fortunate and keeps alive, he will be forever in love. This alone is to be alive to the extremities."

"Man is but the place where I stand. The prospect hence is infinite."

"The well have no time to be sick."

Contents

Chapter	Page
Introduction	1
1. Nutrition	4
2. Supplements	16
3. Detox	32
4. Oxygen	52
5. Diagnostics	60
6. Therapeutics	62
7. Corruption	68
8. Rife	72
9. Spectrochrome	76
10. Bioacoustics	80
11. Attitude	83
12. Regeneration	86
Closing	93
General Attack Plan	97
About the Author	

Introduction

Welcome to the world of natural healing self-empowerment.

In the course of reading this book, you will learn a wide variety of intensely powerful, extremely cost-effective methods to combat a broad diversity of health problems, from mild conditions like skin problems to major diseases such as cancer and AIDS. The information presented here comes from one of the most inspiring groups of science detectives in all history, and includes the writings and findings of qualified medical and naturopathic doctors, humble researchers, and sometimes just from people who give a hoot; even so, any who choose to act on this information should understand that they do so at their own risk, and that reading this information should not supersede seeking the advice of trained professionals, apparently even if they have a dismal track record of failure, and these methods succeed phenomenally well.

Natural healing methods, as defined here, are like notes in a scale that harmonize with the music of nature, and these notes would differ from western medicine's drug approach to solving problems, commonly referred to as drugs for all the bugs, pills for all the ills, as these would be notes that are more like noise than harmony. Technically nature does include even drugs-but we want to focus here mainly on those methods that resonate best with nature's patterns-and drugs rarely do so. Traditionally in the allopathic, or drug-based, approach, some natural plant is stripped down to its parts, one part is labeled as a primary active ingredient, then slightly altered so that wealthy companies may patent their new Frankenstein drug for profit. Alas, as the book *Racketeering In Medicine* by James P. Carter suggests, 80-90% of such drugs may be ineffective.

Today, in 2004, more people have become disillusioned with the failures of the drug companies and their puppets. Dr. Joel Wallach, in his text *Rare Earths: Forbidden*

1

Cures, offers a grim portrait of the allopaths' failures, for during their reign, as detailed in an early 90's study by the World Health Organization, the US ranked 17th in longevity, 19th in healthfulness, and lower still in other health categories when compared to other industrialized nations, and these ranks worsened over time, despite health care industry costs escalating to over a trillion dollars. In addition, Wallach mentions the study by Dr. Sidney Wolfe which shows that a staggering 300,000 people are killed each year due to hospital negligence. As if all this were not bad enough, the average allopath dies at age 58, showing that a pricey education, degrees with elaborate calligraphy on them and years of fancy schooling apparently do nothing to make the allopath smarter than the average weekend warrior at a hockey game. Thusly discouraged, at the moment a higher percentage of people are turning to traditional natural methods that go back decades, if not centuries or even millennia, rather than giving drugs another chance.

Among the methods we shall consider here are nutritional approaches and supplements, detoxifying the organs of detoxification, oxygen therapies, special diagnostic and therapeutic tools, Rife frequency machines, Spectrochrome light therapy, the Bioacoustics of Sharry Edwards, and a brand new body regeneration formula. At the close of the book a general attack plan to wipe out all health problems is offered. Whether anyone can remain sick while following it remains to be seen....

Due to the shortness of this book, there is not space enough to cover each of these areas in overwhelming detail, nor is there time to list all of the problems that can be solved by each pioneer mentioned. The truth is most individuals in this book did such outstanding work the list of illnesses each can beat is simply too vast to mention. If you want to know if a given method can solve a given problem, consult the reference material provided for each pioneer. The only reason cancer is mentioned so often in this book is because for some it is still held up as an unbeatable fate.

While the reader will be more than capable of knowing exactly what to do and where to go to solve a great many health problems after absorbing this book, it is to be hoped that additional research will be done by reading the suggested books and visiting the offered websites for further details—they are all waiting for you when you want them.

Some of you may be familiar with fragments of what nature can offer—but this book intends to offer a more fundamental and complete portrait of the possibilities than ever before.

You can think of this book as a pop-up book, where the pop-ups only happen when you wish to know more on a subject and choose to explore in greater depth using the additional free resources as given. The book itself is simply the core of excellence at the heart of everyone's research—direct and stripped of superfluity. For those who are facing serious health crises and are already drained of cash, it will be difficult to complain about the cost of doing supplementary research when one utilizes libraries that regularly feature free books and free internet access-which is the intention here.

When searching for information on the web, the search engines at google.com and dogpile.com are recommended. To search for information using keywords, simply type in the keywords and hit enter. If you are searching for two keywords that are definitely tied to one another, as in, say, "oxygen therapies", type the words enclosed in quotation marks to cut down on impertinent results. All websites are presumed to begin with http://www unless otherwise indicated. If some of the books mentioned are not in your library system, please consider the department of the library called interlibrary loan, where helpful librarians will seek the book from other libraries nearly always for free, going to neighboring states if necessary. Of course, most books can be purchased as well if necessary, at your local bookstores.

OK, everyone ready?
Here we go.

1. Nutrition

We begin at the beginning, with nutrition. As Amazon John of the Amazon Herb Company states, as he travelled up the Amazon River and become increasingly removed from civilization, he found that the diseases of civilization disappeared.

He is not alone in attributing such health to sound health customs that include proper nutrition. Another individual whose presence may well be forever enmeshed in the subject of nutrition and physical degeneration would be Dr. Weston Price, one of the most outstanding, if still unjustly obscure, researchers in history, and author of the monumental book *Nutrition and Physical Degeneration* first published in 1939. Perhaps a trifle too tired of laboratory research that peevishly looks at one little variable when reality is always grandly multivariable, Price, once head of the American Dental Association, abandoned the classroom for the larger university that is planet Earth, in search of people anywhere who were robustly healthy, to learn the methods of their success. Thus did he travel to a remote village in the Swiss Alps, the peaty reaches of Ireland, the oceanic stretches of Melanesia and Polynesia; chatted with hardy North American Indians, and receptively considered the ideas of spearthrowing Africans. He ventured high into the Andes to learn the wisdom of the Peruvians, and examined thousands of skulls, ancient and modern, examining the arches of the jaws and cross-referencing the data with evidence regarding foods eaten. So what were his conclusions?

The main conclusion was as simple as it was inescapable: wherever the modern diet of refined white flour foods, refined sugar foods, refined salt, polished rice and canned goods appeared, there too could one find poorly formed dental arches, crowded, rotting teeth, narrow nasal passages that in severe cases forced their owners to excessive mouth breathing, correspondingly narrow eye sockets that some have correlated to hampered vision, women with narrow hips that created a great strain on childbearing, and virtually the entire array of modern diseases to boot. His work, and the supplemental work done by Dr. Francis Pottenger, cast serious doubt on the currently prevalent position that all is genetics. Price showed repeatedly that parents with excellent teeth could raise children in the next generation with rotting ones, provided that those children would eat the wondrously barren foods upon which Westerners can never seem to spend enough lavish advertising.

As an experiment demonstrating the prime importance of nutrition, a pig was deprived of vitamin A. The offspring of that pig were born blind with eyes barely formed, if formed at all. Before one could shout genetics, the pig was then given adequate vitamin A, and the next generation of pigs was born with fully functional eyes. Repeatedly and endlessly, problems attributed confidently to genetics simply disappear with adequate nutrition.

The incidence of tooth decay among those eating modern foods versus primitive natural foods was astronomical. Tooth decay was often less than half of a percent among primitive people eating pristine foods, while the exuberant white missionaries trying desperately to educate those unruly savages featured mouths with at least 40 times as much rot, and sometimes worse by orders of magnitude so vast that they might require a very memory rich calculator for computation.

Dr. Francis Pottenger did work that neatly complements the work of Price, work described in the groundbreaking book *Pottenger's Cats*. As Pottenger reveals, cats raised on cooked meat and pasteurized milk (in which enzymes are destroyed) showed smaller skulls, longer legs with more brittle bones, and so many health problems that in the end they would simply die out after a mere 3 generations or so. In contrast, cats raised on raw milk and raw meat were in excellent health. The doctor could reverse the nutritional damage, but it tended to take four generations to undo the harm from cooked foods. The implications for man were clear.

In humans, Pottenger noted that breastfeeding led to more beautiful faces, as the muscles involved pulled the bones into proper shape, where bottle fed babies had narrower cheekbone widths and weaker jaws. Breastfeeding beyond 3 months seemed clearly recommended. Marvin Harris, anthropologist and author of *Our Kind*, argues that breastfeeding might profitably be continued as late as the 2nd year. He is not alone, as the following link shows: http://www.kellymom.com/bf/bfextended/ebf-benefits.html. The better fed the mother, and the more breastfeeding, the better shaped the face, and even the higher the IQ as countless scientists have testified. Dr. Pottenger echoes the views of Price on raw nutrients and hip widths in women, stating an ancient case of Vikings who were completely wiped out because they refused to eat the raw foods of the natives when they arrived in Greenland. The resulting narrow, twisted pelvic girdles were inadequate for childbirth. While Price describes child labor without pain for those well nourished, Pottenger describes the onset of adult teeth without blood or pain in those well nourished.

Imagine what life could be...

At the present day, there exists the Weston Price foundation, websites at westonaprice.org, along with price-pottenger.org, attempting to carry on the tradition of these brave pioneers. We shall be offering some thoughts taken from the current president, Sally Fallon, later in our book, and more on the definition of healthy foods as defined by Price in a moment. The website http://www.4radiantlife.com/ also has further details on related subjects.

Albert Schweitzer, the famous doctor who did volunteer work in Africa, also noted that as the natives began eating modern foods, they also soon acquired modern diseases. While some may still debate whether food has any impact on health, still another man for whom there was no longer any doubt on the subject was the great nutritional pioneer Max Gerson, MD, certified by the American Medical Association, and arguably, the only man who has documented cases of curing cancer through nutrition (one of his most famous patients being Schweitzer himself, though Schweitzer was not treated for cancer). Gerson wrote a book documenting his cancer cases and studies (*A Cancer*

Therapy), and his daughter Charlotte, who has also written a book of her own called *The Gerson Therapy,* additionally has a website at gerson.org.

Thus having whetted our appetite, as it were, on the subject of nutrition, we may now anxiously ask: what exactly do we need from our food according to these and other experts, and what is the best way to get it? Specifically, we need enzymes to maximize efficiency of biochemical reactions, carbohydrates for energy, essential fatty acids for bodily construction of hormones, cells and more, a decent amount of useful proteins for overall structure, and vitamins and minerals. This combination makes for what we shall call *complete nutrition.* So let us combine the ideas of the aforementioned experts to learn more about the best ways to obtain these elements of ultimate vitality.

One idea that all seem to agree on from the beginning is that refined sugar is detrimental. Sugar can have an inflammatory effect and inhibit mineral absorption, not to mention the havoc created in the body system overall. For 87 reasons why refined sugar is bad, please type in this internet link: http://users.kua.net/-haselden/page51e.html. Sugar in the raw state is actually not so bad, as Price recounted stories of sugar plantation owners getting tooth decay and diabetes from their products, while the workers in the field eating the raw sugar cane laden with natural enzymes and other raw goodies, had fine teeth. If many would argue that today it is too hard to find raw sugar, consider using xylitol products instead. This sweet substance (occurring naturally in raspberries, strawberries and plums) not only substitutes for sugar, but has a track record of helping tooth enamel, according to *Nexus* magazine. It also can force *candida* to slide out of the body rather than maintain its grip as it can when fed refined sugar. See the websites at xylitolnow.com or vrp.com for more, or see the *Nexus* article. Stevia was also featured in *Nexus* as a sugar alternative.

In the Gerson therapy, fresh organic fruit and vegetable juices, a quality source of carbohydrates and vitamins, are at the heart. Why are these juices so important? For starters,

7

95% of the essential nutrition of plants is hidden in the juice. The remaining fiber, while good for passing the bowel contents, is not directly essential for nutrition. Gerson found that, in the cases of those with advanced illness, it would be more profitable to take the juice from three carrots and combine that with other nutrients, rather than have someone eat three whole carrots and then be stuffed. Most importantly, these fresh juices still contain viable enzymes, most of which can be weakened when heated to about 118 degrees F, and destroyed at 130 degrees, making cooking a damaging act.

Intact enzymes not only aid the body in food digestion, they also relieve the body of a burden to produce its own enzymes from the liver, pancreas and spleen. Once relieved of these burdens, the organs are better able to maintain overall health. The importance of this point can hardly be exaggerated, and the full case is sharply made in the *tour de force* opus of Dr. Edward Howell, *Food Enzymes for Health and Longevity*. Dr. Howell equates enzymes with nothing less than the essence of life itself. Enzymes also can be crucial to maintaining the cleanliness of the bowel, whose state, as we shall see, largely determines the fate of the rest of the body.

For those who do cook, microwave cooking should be avoided. Two articles that explore the background of this subject may be found at the following links: http://www.alkalizeforhealth.net/Lmicrowaveovens.htm and http://www.nexusmagazine.com/articles/microwave.html

One may also survey the alkalize for health site, http://www.alkalizeforhealth.net/ for more info on many subjects mentioned here.

Juices also contain proteins, vitamins and minerals in an ideally bioavailable form, meaning that the body can use these nutrients far more easily than factory made equivalents (note that protein in meat may be more abundant, but only 1/3 can be used according to Carlson Wade, as the body has a hard time breaking down protein in this form into its constituent amino acids—at least without additional enzymatic help). Cheap centrifugal juicers do work for this application, although with limited benefits. Consult the Gerson therapy for juicer recommendations. It should be noted that juicing may be more indicated in extreme cases of illness, and that healthy individuals should never overlook the importance of natural fiber--one would never want to juice to such an extent that all fiber is eliminated from the diet, as the consequences for the bowels can be extreme. We shall return to bowel health shortly. To be sure, the Gersons never overlooked the importance of fiber. One raw carrot a day is an excellent source of fiber, and is ideal for binding toxins in the intestine and moving them along. Nuts and grains from organic trail mixes (note that Dr. Howell discourages the consumption of unsprouted nuts and seeds as they contain enzyme inhibitors— sprouting ones are enzyme rich) can also move food along and maintain a quick bowel transit time, which can be crucial to maintaining overall health. Fresh, whole grain breads made with sea salt can be excellent sources of fiber.

Another key point in Gerson therapy is that ill people tend to have elevated levels of sodium, while being low in potassium. Eating regular helpings of organic baked potatoes (without refined salt and in some cases without salt altogether), bananas and fresh tomatoes can help restore potassium levels and the natural balance. Dr. West's research sheds more light on this elevated sodium level—claiming that it is caused by excess levels of the blood proteins albumin, globulin and fibrinogen, which in turn are caused from excessive animal protein consumption (without enzymes). For more details on this process, check out this link: http://www.omarstouch.com/htdocs/goldenseven.htm

All of these researchers agree that fat, in the right form, is also essential. The 3 types we humans use are called omega 3, omega 6, and omega 9. The 9s can be built from the 3s and 6s. Most foods in the stores are preserved with fats of the omega 6 hydrogenated variety to add shelf life, but this form of hydrogenated oil fat (just check labels for hydrogenated oil) is tough for the body to process, and overloads the body with omega 6 fatty acids. The ratio of omega 6 to omega 3 should be ideally about 2 to 1, but because of the omega 6 craze ends up being at least about 10:1 for many if not most people on a Western diet. By taking supplements of two teaspoons of flaxseed or borage oil a day, such as Barlean's, the omega 3 fatty acids can be restored to normal levels. These fats are vital to the myelin sheath insulation in brain cells, and in some cases, children with attention deficit disorders have become normal simply by eating a correct balance of fatty acids, as described in the book called *The Omega Plan* by Artemis Semopoulous. These fatty acids are also linked to prostaglandins, which regulate pain. A better fatty acid balance can thus minimize some forms of pain, menstrual pain being an example that often sees benefits from fatty acid balancing.

The oil also assists the nutrients in fruit and vegetable juices to be absorbed even more efficiently, as Gerson therapy attests. Fats are further used as comforting padding between joints, and are also integral to many cell membranes— which is evidenced easily by the description of their structure— phospholipid bilayers—where lipid means fat. They are not called essential fatty acids for nothing!

The nutritional evidence from several sources agrees on the bountiful benefits of fresh organic produce juiced for maximum benefit, or consumed uncooked, with flaxseed or borage oil supplementation.

Lita Lee, in her book, *The Enzyme Cure,* also speaks of a few other fatty acid oils that may be consumed safely, such as coconut oil. Fresh coconut oil apparently has a great many health benefits-in one case, a man recovered from AIDS simply by consuming large quantities of fresh coconut oil (See book below for more on this story)(see Radiant Life link above or moonlight health link below for how to get some). For more on coconut oil, see the March/April 2002 issue of *Nexus* magazine, or the entire book *The Healing Miracles of Coconut Oil* by Bruce Fife (Fife notes excellent dental development in those who commonly consumed coconut). You may also wish to read up on many of these health topics as reported at the Nexus magazine main site, at nexusmagazine.com. For example, an article archived there called

The Oiling Of America by the aforementioned Sally Fallon goes into the fatty acid oil issue in much greater detail than we can present here. Much of this new research portrays socalled trans fatty acids, or acids with a chemical structure featuring carbons on opposite sides of the main chemical chain, as harmful, while the unbranched ones are more beneficial. The research also questions the prevalent notion that saturated fats in and of themselves are villains-see the Price website for more.

Charlotte Gerson does raise a good point on the subject of changing the rules of her approach. She says that whenever anyone tries to offer nutritional advice to a cancer patient that conflicts with the Gerson therapy, ask them how many cancer cases they have cured-and that usually shuts them up. Not to say that Lita Lee is wrong with her fatty acid oil recommendations, mind you, but that most rules in these therapies are strict, and when you are trying to save a life, it is not wise to fool with nature's rules by taking advice from those who have not witnessed success. Since Lita Lee has seen success, her ideas are worth considering.

Price himself is another who has seen decisive success with his rules, and he became a rather unequivocal champion of natural butter, and milk, consumed *with its fat*, in the natural state. The process of pasteurization, or extreme heating, may kill bacteria and viruses, but it is also enzyme slaughter, severely hampering the absorption of nutrients. Homogenization, the process of dispersing fat evenly through the milk for a smoother consistency, also warps nature's perfectly designed original plan, and further interferes with nutrient absorption.

For those who complain that everyone means well, and that if these processes like pasteurization were abandoned all dairy products could become deadly, we should point out that none of these foods would suffer if they were preserved with food grade hydrogen peroxide (as a small amount of milk actually is preserved on the store shelves) and that if you simply raised the cows with proper care, they would not get contaminated with such nasty pathogens to begin with. There is much debate on milk, but little

11

attention paid to the specific points just addressed, and until they are addressed, the debate will continue to suffer.

We have seen at this point that we can get carbohydrates from fruits and vegetables, and fats from sources such as flaxseed, borage, tropical oils and dairy, but what of proteins?

Hardcore athletic types in the gym may have heard the suggested ratio of consumed carbs:fats:proteins should be 40%/30%/30%, and that overall protein intake should be 1 gram of protein /1 lb. lean body weight/day-so that a 160 pound man should be consuming 160 grams of protein per day. Another scientist argues that half that amount should be used-so that the 160 pound man should consume 80 grams of protein per day-who is right?

According to C. Samuel West, both men are wrong, and very wrong at that. Dr. West believes, based on his experiences and reported in *The Golden 7 Plus 1*, that the ideal ratio of carbs/fat/proteins should actually be 80/10/10, and that overall protein consumption of 25 to 30 grams of protein per day, such as one could get even from fruits and vegetables, is enough for even a hardcore athlete. He maintains that strength and body structure will not suffer but even be better for the lowered protein intake. Further, during the most phenomenal growth of the human lifetime, that which occurs during infancy, mother's milk is the primary nutrition, and that milk usually contains less than 2% protein, and the infant can double in size on such sustenance. Followers of West cite Olympic medalists and even bodybuilding champions who were vegetarians as examples of tough customers with relatively lower protein intakes. See the following link for a deeper discussion: http://www.all-creatures.org/cb/aprotein.html

Nature herself offers strong oxen as examples of vegetarians, and scientists have cited the example of our close cousins the gorillas as indicators of the diet best for man. The clear rule appears to be that, generally speaking, cooked meat is not healthy for man. By considering the anatomical evidence, such as teeth structure, length of the intestinal tract, and eating habits of our nearest relatives in the animal kingdom, it is easy to see that man was built to eat plant food, and we eat meat at our own risk. Do further research into the findings of Dr. West on this subject to learn more.

Stanley Burroughs adds an additional cautionary note, warning that the stomach lining is protected by sodium, and that meat pulls this sodium away, thereby weakening the stomach walls. Worse still, today's modern meats, coming from cows raised on a terrible diet which may include road kills, plastic flea collar remains, and other horrors, may reach us loaded with pesticides, drugs from the water supply, and antibiotics, not to mention strange hormones whose effects are uncertain.

Another note of potential value for the alert is the idea that particle size influences absorbability as a general rule, such that proteins in fluid form absorb faster and cause less troublesome work for the body than larger, clumpier ones. Thus form of protein as well as quantity may have a significant effect.

Not long ago, an article appeared in *Nexus* magazine attempting a comprehensive annihilation of all arguments supporting vegetarianism. This article does not deal grapple either with West's research or with the crucial subject of minerals, and thus the article is decidedly shallow at best.

West and others like him question not only whether meat is necessary, but they complain of countless known hazards from excessive protein consumption. You can start to form a picture of this by reading the article linked here: http://www.nutrigenesis.com/WLprotein_dangers.htm. A list of dangers from too high protein intake includes: production of high ammonia levels, liver and kidney damage, rotting matter in the intestines which can host countless parasites, bacteria and viruses bent on our destruction, and trapped plasma proteins which clog cell gates and prevent vital oxygen and water from nourishing cells. This last point was critical to West's pioneering work, and was reinforced in the writings of Dr. John Whitman Ray, who spoke similarly of mucoproteins clogging cell gates from high protein consumption. Those who favor high protein, low carb diets

13

for the sake of losing weight may be causing more damage than helping themselves.

But what about those crazy Eskimos? Did Dr. Howell not report that they ate 10 pounds of animal flesh a day without incident? Yes, he did, but *they ate the flesh raw*, like Pottenger's cats. As long as the enzymes break down the food, apparently you can get away with large protein amounts up to a point. If you are weak or by some reasonable standard low on muscle mass, boost protein levels only by accompanying them with protein digesting enzymes. Lymph node pain (armpit or groin for example), gut pain and flatulence after a heavy protein meal are often signs of undigested food, so either consume less protein or increase supplemental enzymes.

An easy way to settle the matter individually is urinalysis. If your urine shows too high a protein level, then simply cut back on animal proteins. If your fingernails show vertical striations, gently nudge protein, vitamin, and mineral intake higher until the nails become smooth.

Though cooked meat has its hazards, not all plants are good for us. Many believe soy to be beneficial, for example, but a closer look at the evidence suggests this is a dubious conclusion. Soy contains substances that can adversely affect hormones, and cause several other problems. Consult the article archived at the *Nexus* site, on the dangers of soy foods for more.

And while meat may not be such an ideal source of protein, other animal sources of protein, like the aforementioned dairy, and free range eggs, may be used safely in most cases. If you cannot get raw dairy, but can get milk free of hormones, pesticides, antibiotics and the rest, it might be useful in limited quantities, with enzymes, even if pasteurized and homogenized—but strive for raw. We know these industries suffer from numerous faults, but why not press them to improve standards rather than abandon a potentially pivotal source of nutrition?

Given the variations in individuals, and the variations in the goals of an individual at different times, there is no ideal ratio of proteins to carbs to fats applicable to all men at all times. When you need more energy, eat more carbs. When you need less, eat less. When you need more muscle mass, stronger hair and nails, or to repair digestive tract linings or protein tissues, eat more protein. If you are heading for gout, or experience the aforementioned high protein woes, cut back. If your weight is ideal, find the minimum protein you need to maintain this level of strength. If your weight drops, you have gone too far. If you are overweight with undigested fat, increase lipase, the fat digesting enzyme, or other fat digesting enzymes, or add garlic, until the fat is gone. If your joints are creaking, your skin shows dangerously low body fat, or you have any woes associated with low fat or the wrong fat, boost flax oil, coconut oil, dairy cream, or the fatty oil of your enlightened choice.

Thus do we cover the main body of proper nutrition, but given the nutritional emptiness of most foods, supplements may be needed. We tackle these next, starting with one of the most important of supplements, minerals.

2. Supplements

Minerals are not tackled with much depth in health discussions, and what an enormously important subject to neglect! Can you imagine a man who had noted that all the diseases of humans were suffered by other animals, and who then learned a simple way to wipe out all these diseases in animals? Can you imagine that same man being fired from his job when he proposed the comprehensive plan to wipe out the diseases of man? Then you can imagine the life of Dr. Joel Wallach. His simple way of wiping out disease? Making sure that animals received proper minerals.

Sure, minerals pop up in a perfunctory, bland way in discussions of health, but how many times have you heard that minerals come in three basic forms: inorganic, chelated and plant derived colloidal? Most minerals sold in stores are inorganic, with an absorption rate of about 8-12%. Those minerals chelated or bound to amino acids can have an absorption rate of about 40%. Plant derived colloidal (colloidal can be understood here as very small particle-sized) minerals feature absorption rates as high as 100%, and are mostly in the 95-100% range. What kind of impact can this have on your health? A miraculous one.

It is interesting to note how many health authorities speak so sagely to us while looking out from bodies with unimproving grey hair and sometimes no hair at all-which would not be so bad if these were not signs of mineral deficiency, and thus scientific ignorance! Dr. Wallach helped establish the bar when it comes to mineral deficiency, and gives us quite a list of minerals and their functions in the body. We have time to hit on only highlights here, but for a fuller story read his thick text *Rare Earths: Forbidden Cures*, or consult his website at majesticearth-minerals.com. Dr. Wallach found chromium and vanadium lacking in diabetics, for example, and that when these minerals were eventually restored to normal levels, the diabetes vanished. Cancer was mostly a case of selenium deficiency. Blood vessel elasticity, skin elasticity (and breast lift) and hair color were regulated chiefly by copper, while hearing and hair growth were significantly influenced by tin. Zinc plays a profound role in immunity and was often found lacking in those with Down's syndrome, while arsenic and boron play key roles in bone maintenance. The list goes on and on. For our purposes, we would like to point out several items: First, the reasons for the high absorption rates of colloidal minerals are: that the particle size is extremely small, is oppositely charged the lining of the digestive tract for quick absorption, and is in an organic form more friendly to the body. Second, one does not have to buy a zillion supplements to get all mineral benefits, but can get them all in one fell swoop, in complete formulations such as 75 Colloidal Minerals, Liquid Logic and Liquid Life (the latter two include vitamins and amino acid and herbal complexes in differing concentrations) from the Rockland Corporation at reachforlife.com or 1-800-258-5028 (please mention this book and number 21548 if you call--the mention can help further this research). Here you have 70 odd plant derived minerals at once, with a spectacular track record going all the way back to pioneer days when mineral baths worked wonders.

A recommended maintenance dose is 8 tsp/loz/100lbs body weight/day. However, as most people are mineral deficient a kickstart dose (twice the maintenance dose) may be recommended until such time as the body is on track. More specifically, a loose recommendation might be kickstart one month if under 30 or with no evident health problems, kickstart 2 months if between 30 and 60 or with a moderate health problem, and kickstart 3 months if over 60 or with a serious problem. One can of course drop to maintenance dose when the health problems disappear, or whenever you like for that matter.

You can even exceed the kickstart dose if you have the money, inclination and constitution. Sometimes the body begins to detox when minerals are started, and this can be tough if one has a lot of garbage to get rid of. If you detox immediately after starting minerals and do not feel so hot at first, you may wish to delay your kickstart dose until you feel your body is ready for it, perhaps waiting a week or two. Also note that if you take too much, your bowel contents may liquefy (because of too high magnesium), leading to a mild diarrhea—nothing dangerous, but not nice. If any doubt the sheer power of these minerals and demand proof, use them instead of rock dust in the experiment below!! So does one need to supplement with minerals for the rest of a lifespan? If you want to stay young and healthy, the answer is yes, you will have to get your minerals from somewhere, because *our bodies are designed to run on these things*! But why, one may ask, is our food so mineral deficient to being with?

Elmer Heinrich, in the *Root of All Disease* sold by Rockland, answers this question. The bottom line is: the international conglomerates simply use brainless ways of growing food. It seems that someone once made a comparison between a plant grown with no minerals to one grown with 3 minerals based in nitrogen, phosphorus and potassium, (also known as NPK) and then strangely concluded that these 3 mineral types were all a plant needed-WRONG! Plants need tons of minerals, as we do. They can make their own vitamins and even enzymes, but the plants rely on whatever soil they are grown on for minerals, and thanks to silly farming techniques which flout ancient wisdom regarding crop rotation, hydration and other technical matters, the plants suffer greatly. The evidence for this is easy enough to gather for yourself. Grow some plants yourself, the right way, and prove what is possible! The right way, in this case, would be to grow those plants with rock dust, granite rock dust being the best found thus far. Grind the rock to a fine powder, then sprinkle liberally in the soil, and let the plants do their thing. The vital trace minerals will be greedily seized by plant roots, and monstrously healthy plants will result. As you may doubt your own eyes, it is a simple matter to conduct a scientific experiment, fertilizing one plant with dust and another any way you like. You might not want to plant the rock dust plant in your favorite pot though. Sometimes the growth rate is so intense even a large pot may crack from the thunderous growth.

"Nasty" insects, contrary to popular belief, nearly always attack only unhealthy plants, and will leave hardy ones alone, just like wild wolves are not careless predators of caribou, but actually strengthen the herds by weeding out the old and weak. Pesticides not only kill insects needlessly, but also harm helpful bacteria attempting to nourish plant roots. Even weeds, according to Dr. Phil Callahan, are not the evil commonly imagined, but tend to manifest as desperation measures assisting minerals on the way up from soil depths should that soil be lacking in nutrients. Should you do a rock dust plant growth experiment, the man you will eventually want to thank for this insight is a fellow by the name of Julius Hensel (for more background, see http://www.agrowinn.com/bread-stones.htm). He may not be the first to observe this phenomenon, but he has done much to popularize it.

Anyone who opts to grow veggies should further consult the popular text *How To Grow More Vegetables* by John Jeavons to learn skills that enable your yields to be 2 to 6 times greater than the produce of our so-called agricultural revolution. Clean water, oxygenrich water, magnetized water, and vortexed water can all further influence plant growth rates.

Now imagine, if a plant is growing that well, and beams with such radiant health, what do you think you will be like when you eat the fruits and vegetables of that plant, or juice them? Boggles the mind.

Thus one way we could all avoid supplements is to grow our own food, or buy from those who grow it correctly.

Otherwise, if you want the benefits, supplement with minerals.

A distinction is often made between the major minerals and the trace minerals. The major minerals, as their name suggests, serve overtly crucial functions in the body, and while this insight is impressed upon the average medical student, the public should be just as informed on this subject. Though the members in the major minerals group varies according to source, many would say that there are seven major minerals: calcium, magnesium, phosphorus, potassium, sodium, chloride, and sulfur.

Many of these minerals, in an ionized form, form what are known as electrolytes—they are the carriers of electrical energy and information in our bodies, and as such have a drastic impact on our health. Those who are athletic are likely to drain off their body's store of electrolytes, and it was this theory that lay behind the development of certain sports drinks. Athletes depleted of electrolytes would down these drinks during games, and restore lost energy—and win games. Yet nature has always had her own preferred methods of supplying these major minerals. Raw milk is an excellent source of virtually all major minerals. Even sulfur is present in the form of methylsulfonylmethane—or msm. Bananas are also an excellent major mineral supplier. Check foods for major mineral content!

Since intense physical activity puts a strain on the major minerals, it behooves athletes to get ahead of the burden they will be placing on themselves by loading up on them in advance of strenuous activity. Those who like to exercise, for example, will find their workouts far more profitable if they load up on calcium, magnesium and potassium ahead of time. Such a ready source of electrolytes in the blood will greatly enhance the workouts.

Since Dr. Robert Becker showed in his books *The Body Electric* and *Cross Currents* that the meridian system described in acupuncture/acupressure actually carries DC analog electricity, and the major minerals are carriers of electricity, it then follows that the entire energy meridian system can be revitalized when at low power simply by restoring the levels of major minerals. The body can conserve sodium, but not potassium. The majority of people consume too many phosphates. Thus scientists have formulated a specific major mineral supplement: cal/mag/potass/ boron (calcium/magnesium/ potassium/boron) to target the minerals most likely to be needed (boron helps to stabilize the levels of calcium and magnesium). This supplement is available at Rockland and elsewhere, and is fantastic for maintaining or replenishing vital major minerals. Note again that excessive magnesium intake may liquefy bowel contents.

There are a host of problems that may well be wiped off the face of the earth when mastery of major minerals becomes widespread: permanent scars, stretch marks, baldness, teeth with dental fillings, damaged organs. Many of these negative situations occur when dead proteins, or other obstacles, block the flow of electrical energy until such time as the nervous system and the brain lose interest in correcting the trouble area, and the information flow is cut off. Yet if the information flow is restored, the flaw can vanish.

This analysis is similar to that described in "body electronics" pioneered by John Whitman Ray, who first prepped his clients with a nutrition regimen essentially identical to the one described in this book, then used acupressure in a special way, with the result that many permanent scars disappeared. In some cases metal dental fillings fell out, and this makes sense when the ideas presented in Hansen's *Key to Ultimate Health* are additionally considered.

According to Hansen, energy meridians flow directly to the teeth, and fillings block the energy flow. It would thus be logical if Ray's acupressure methods created a surge of energy through a blocked meridian, such that a filling might eventually be ejected. Yet it also follows that mere restoration of major minerals should eventually accomplish the same task without spending hundreds if not thousands of dollars seeking special help.

This explains why the article linked here: (http://www.rawpaleodiet.org/dental-regeneration-1.html) notes that metal fillings were often ejected by those supplementing specifically with cal/mag/potass/boron.

The subject of body regeneration will be tackled in fuller detail in the chapter devoted to the subject.

Sulfur, the last of the major minerals, deserves special mention. Though Dr. Wallach argues that copper is critical to hair color, there is absolutely no mistaking the fact that grey hair will disappear when adequate *sulfur* levels are restored. Nature's richest sources of sulfur are garlic and onions. For those interested in a supplement, Rockland offers Garlic Oil Triple Strength and Odorless Garlic. Amounts taken per individual can vary—some can take the recommended dose, or 2, 3 or 4 times that if their body wishes for it.

It is fascinating to note that certain individuals cough and detox when garlic is used to restore their hair color—as if the body is getting rid of the toxins that damage hair color. Could it be that heavy metals that can be chelated by garlic (see next section) are hurting our hair cells? Garlic taken with proteins has an amazing ability to aid the detox process of the body. For more on this subject see this link: http://www.healingdaily.com/detoxification-diet/garlic.htm. Not for nothing is garlic considered the king of the herbs.

Sulfur is also one of the major elements comprising our proteins, along with carbon, hydrogen, oxygen and nitrogen.

These major minerals are of prime importance, so make sure you get enough of them, and also of the major and minor trace minerals.

It should be mentioned that there are some slimy types claming to sell colloidal minerals out there, but who are pretty much lying in their product representations-buyer beware!

Many who have restored minerals to their normal levels have regrown hair. By taking formulations such as Rockland's Body Booster orally and/or dabbing the minerals on the head, hair has regrown. Those who take oxygen supplements, like those described later, regrow hair even faster. Those who add in 5 alpha reductase enzyme inhibitors, such as those cheaply available in saw palmetto, improve faster still. Those who clean up any dental tooth metal can also speed up the process (thus chelation, too, explained below, can aid in this process), as can those who exercise to get the blood flowing. Enzymes (see below) are an additional pivotal speed factor. Note that hair follicles inactive for many years may have trouble rejuvenating due to cross linked fibrous proteins near the base of the hair. A method (hinted at above) to solve this problem has now been devised, and appears in the body regeneration chapter!

As for restoring hair color, while sulfur helps in this task, restoring copper helps also. Take formulations like 75 Colloidal Minerals or Liquid Life (while obeying the rest of the nutrition recommendations given here) and watch color begin to return in 60 to 90 days. For still better absorption, take the copper with the amino acids tyrosine and phenylalanine (sold at health food stores and also sold cheaply at Rockland's reachforlife.com website). Enzyme supplements are strongly recommended in this process. Chelation also can have a significant impact on restoring hair color, and in some cases may be absolutely essential to prime the body to receive the benefit of quality nutrients that affect hair color. In the cases of both regrowing hair and restoring color, again please try to minimize refined sugar intake.

Always remember the combination of vitamins, minerals and enzymes is necessary for most reactions to flourish in the body. For example, vitamin A, whether in its whole form retinol or precursor carotenoid form (note: you can supposedly toxically overdose on retinol, but if you take the building blocks of vitamin A—precursors like the beta carotene in carrots, or the carotenoids of tomatoes—the body will build only as much vitamin A as necessary without overdoing it), along with B vitamins, plays a key role in hair color and health—those who overlook vitamins and focus only on minerals will improve far more slowly than those who have all three elements of the critical trio.

A note on doses of minerals and vitamins is in order for any who have not read Dr. Harold Rosenberg's *Doctor's Book of Vitamin Therapy*. As annoying as it may be, *you* are the ultimate authority on your own doses. As recounted in the book, the variation among individuals is far too wild for anyone to take charts recommending doses for all very seriously. Especially in instances where one has been vitamin or mineral deficient for long periods, the doses necessary to reset the body may end up being extreme. Cases abound of those whose situations only improved at

50 times a given recommended vitamin or mineral dose. Your body can give you the clues you need—if you do not trick it with garbage food (described above in the Price nutrition info). Natural cravings (unlike cravings for processed foods which trick your taste buds into believing certain nutrients are present when they are not) guide you to find the vitamins, minerals and enzymes you need, so listen to them. Your body will tell you what it needs. Even so, make no mistake, the critical and often unsung combination of vitamins, minerals and enzymes needs all three players to tango— virtually any health initiative neglecting the whole is doomed to total or partial failure. Watch to see that capsules are favored over tablets in most supplement situations—the binders and fillers in tablets can be toxic—and never forget, smaller particles means more surface area, faster absorption, and party time for the relieved liver and pancreas.

See why chewing your food is so important now??

Given the importance of minerals, we should not leave this topic without acknowledging the controversial findings of the French scientist Louis Kervran, as reported in his unexpected book, *Biological Transmutations.* According to Kervran, as much as this discovery may make physicists throw their food in public restaurants, bacteria and their enzymes may be capable of transmuting lower elements to higher ones. Kervran describes many experiments by himself and others which demonstrate, for example, that manganese can be converted into iron by the body, and that silica and magnesium can be converted to calcium. These experiments were hardly whimsical and often involved the use of highly sophisticated equipment to assess results. Kervran even went so far as to say that should there be a mineral deficiency (such as one diagnosed by relying on Wallach's data, for example) one may be better off taking a mineral that can be transmuted to the deficient one more than taking the one of which a deficiency is suspected. Crazy as this may sound, it is intriguing to note that Kervran suggests that 2 oxygens = 1 sulfur (16+16=32 for the chemist) and that sulfur is strangely found often with oxygen, and that further, if one considers the evidence, sulfur appears to aid in restoring hair color, and 2 sulfurs = 1 copper (32 + 32 = 64).

Coincidence? If not, what consequences may there be for iron deficiency anemia? Osteoporosis? Hair color restoration? What strategy should one use? A safe path may be to study the transmutations and take minerals in "transmutation teams" (copper with sulfur (methylsulfonylmethane or msm— available from Rockland for example; onions or garlic (Rockland has a triple strength garlic oil)) to restore copper, for example). If we ignore Kervran's findings, we may never know... Yet the safest path, most likely, is to take formulations like 75 colloidal minerals or rock dust grown produce that offer a multitude of choices, and let the body decide what it wants.

If you try a supplement and become nauseous, be aware that it may not be the main ingredient that makes you sick, as much as toxins unwittingly added by the manufacturer. Switch companies to be sure it was not a given brand that made you sick. Many companies have poor standards in quality control of their products. Linus Pauling once traced *all* diseases to mineral deficiencies. In any case, in our currently mineral deficient world, minerals, especially the plant derived colloidal ones, may indeed be the cornerstone of proper nutrition.

And now let us look at what other supplements are most recommended for those for whom life without Sugar Blasted Wacky Poofs is unlivable.

In addition to lifesustaining minerals, if one must persist in such poor eating habits, taking digestive enzymes available in health food stores can help ease the strain of eating frankenfoods tremendously. Most enzymes end with the suffix -ASE. Lipase is a fat digesting enzyme, amylase and disaccharrides are sugar digesting enzymes, protease digests protein, and cellulase digests plant fibers, for example. Bromelain, found in pineapple, digests protein, while papain, the main papaya enzyme, can digest proteins carbs and fats. In fact, papaya and kiwi fruit are the only two fruits known that actually offer a surplus of enzymes—thus they are superb for weight loss and overall health (some say supposedly papaya has abortifacient properties for those to whom that is relevant). One can cater enzymes to the kinds of meals eaten. Enzymes, as described in *Enzymes, The Fountain of Life*, by DA Lopez, perform thousands of vital functions everywhere in the body and can speed up some reaction rates by a factor of at least a thousand. With the right enzymes, we can heal days if not weeks faster. To repeat, Lita Lee has written a book on this subject you may wish to explore, called *The Enzyme Cure*. Using enzymes she has relieved countless diseases and conditions. *The Complete Book of Enzyme Therapy* also has a few things to say on the subject of enzymes. For more on enzymes on the web, visit moonlighthealth.com and get a catalog of enzyme preparations and their multifarious uses.

A cost effective basic digestive enzyme set called Wild Oats Enzyme Complex is sold by Wild Oats (wildoats.com), while Enzyme Plus is sold by the ever alert Rockland, cost $8 (note the Rockland formulation adds hydrochloric acid to aid digestion, which can cause upset stomachs in healthier people, but be of benefit to those whose stomach acids have grown weak). Whole Foods is another national brand with fairly cheap enzymes. American Health's Super Papaya Enzyme Plus is also outstanding, and especially cost effective. A diabetic boy once had blood sugar at 1500. The medical doctors, with all their tools, could not lower his blood sugar below 1200. Yet his blood sugar was normalized by Super Papaya Enzymes—in one week!

Note that some companies list enzyme content by weight, but what you really need to know is the activity level of the enzyme, not its weight, as two enzymes can weigh the same, yet one could be 1,000 times more potent than the other. The standards in this regard have been set in the government's Food Chemical Codex (FCC) listing units like HUT for protease, or LU for Lipase. Alas, different companies may or may not use these units. They may use USP units, BP units, FIP units, EP units, or units of their own imagination. The aforementioned enzymes have worked well for many, but search for the one that works best for you. The goal of enzyme use is not merely to make all bowel movements proportionate to meals (in and of itself a most valiant goal) but to attain that highest of health states wherein the stool is occasionally coated with a beautiful green—the color of healthy bile. When you find this shade on your stool, you may feel you have arrived on the enzyme scene.

Diabetics above all should use enzymes until cured (and then eat only food with complete nutrition thereafter)!

As yet another of nature's gifts, we find that each plant contains enzymes related to its nutrients. Fruits containing fructose, or fruit sugar, have sugar digesting enzymes, while fatty avocados contain fat digesting enzymes (eating cooked meat we get no such helpful assistance). It follows logically that if we eat sugar digesting enzymes with sugary meals, and use similar reasoning with carbohydrates and fats, we best harmonize with nature. Note that bananas, avocados, and mangoes are three of nature's richest enzyme sources according to Dr. Howell. To test enzymes' power, one may wish to prepare several small samples of oatmeal, then place the enzymes you wish to test in each small bowl. If the enzymes work, the food will visibly begin breaking down. You can buy more of whatever enzymes digest the food best.

Still another most crucial supplement would be the intestinal microorganisms. Bacteria have assumed a more and more prominent role in this health research as time goes by. Yes, bacteria can be bad, but they can also be good, and if you hurt the good ones enough—*you die*. In nature, our ancestors ate not only raw fruits and vegetables teeming with minerals, vitamins and enzymes, but also swallowed helpful armies of bacteria that set up shop in our guts and began helping us around the clock, busily manufacturing nutrients for our mutual benefit.

Today, we stupidly chlorinate our water, drinking it, bathing in it, fertilizing soil with it, slaughtering these helpful troops by the millions, with eventual tragic health consequences. Bacterial supplements are available from places like Rockland and can get you on your way. The types of people you would like to see if you could tour your guts would be acidophilus, lactobacillus, chlorella and spirulina (all available from Rockland). Certain green foods may be rich in these groups as well, so check them out. Jennifer Gerhardt, mentioned below, believes homemade sauerkraut is ideal for gut recolonization, as is raw milk if you can find it.

Iodine, which can be taken in many ways, can be another key supplement assisting overall metabolism. The thyroid gland, instrumental to metabolism, relies heavily on iodine, but too much refined salt of the sodium chloride variety can displace the iodine in thyroid compounds. This was observed frequently in the Gerson therapy. Sodium chloride can also act as a general enzyme inhibitor according to DA Lopez and a bacterial gut enemy according to Gerhardt. Refined salt initially had no iodine and the health consequences were disastrous—a situation which led to iodized salt, but natural sea salt is an easier way to get iodine restored. We can get sodium and chloride plentifully without using salt, and if it can hurt our good bacteria, it should be used sparingly if at all. Using Lugol's solution, available from pharmacists and Dr. Hulda Clark for example, is another way to restore depleted iodine. Bear in mind that Dr. Clark, whose work we will explore more fully later, and the Gersons differ on the amount of Lugol's to be taken in different cases, so study each path and use your own judgement. Another way to get iodine is to eat those foods rich in iodine. Who knows but you may develop a love of seaweed out of this. Iodine, being a mineral, is of course included in Rockland's minerals.

The quest for ideal health, for some, lies in fighting off the effects of the aging process. For those who are over forty, and for some under that age with certain problems, melatonin may be the answer. For openers, you may wish to catch up to the story of melatonin as reported by Dr Walter Pierpaoli, in his book *The Melatonin Miracle*. Melatonin is a perfectly natural master regulator hormone, controlling the levels of many other body hormones and maintaining overall balance. It can boost the immune system, restore an imbalanced sleep cycle, rejuvenate the body, enhance the sex drive, influence blood sugar levels, help with menopause symptoms (as does pregnenolone and progesterone creams) and much, much more. Its levels taper with age and synthetic melatonin may restore this balance. It should be taken at night before bed, but taking too much can lead to headaches the next day, and, for some, bad dreams. The recommended dosages are in the book, but one can start with 1 mg and experiment.

Perhaps melatonin would naturally reset its levels if the body was detoxed and given complete nutrition...further research will tell...

Still another realm of supplementation concerns natural herbs. One can get a general overview of herbs and their uses from the back of the book called *The Parasite Menace* by Skye Weintraub. Another text would be *Let's Play Herbal Doctor* by Dr. Wallach. Still another massive overview textbook covering many nutritional topics in addition to herbs is *Prescription for Nutritional Healing* by Balch and Balch. And yet another is available from Rockland: *Homeopathy and Herbs*. A general overall herbal detox is available from Rockland, called Tox-Away, and features garlic, the impressive red clover used by Harry Hoxsey, fenugreek recommended by Dr. Clark, and more. It is yet another strategy to assist overall detox described more fully in the next section.

Garlic is the king of the herbs. It has a track record of success going back thousands of years. Its sulfur (one of the six major minerals) alone has rich benefits to the body (as in restoring hair color as described above, to name one benefit). Garlic can control cholesterol and blood sugar levels, and greatly aid digestion. Rockland at reachforlife.com sells a garlic oil with allicin releasing factor-allicin being the primary active ingredient that makes garlic such a bane for so many pathogens that disturb us. For the gutsy, one could also peel out a clove or garlic, and eat it. Those less gutsy may wish to chop the clove in tiny pieces, let the pieces dissolve a bit in some clean water, then drink the water. *Always sip first to make sure you do not burn your throat.* You can wait a half hour for a mild drink or two hours or more for a more potent one. You can even bathe in the stuff if it is not world series time with your partner in the bedroom. And hey, while we have a moment to mention such activity, how about taking a moment to acknowledge the ideas of Willa Shaffer in her booklet *Wild Yam: Birth Control Without Fear.* She claims that if a woman faithfully uses wild yam extract for 2 months, she can have what appears to be perfect birth control. See the booklet for more. One can also add an additional safety factor by checking saliva with special small microscope instruments-ask health food stores for more on how to check your ovulatory cycle by studying your saliva (test kits are also available from Dr. Chi at this web address: http://www.allfit.com/chiorder3.html, or phone (888- 272-2224)). Other major herbs in addition to garlic and wild yam can include olive leaf extract, grapefruit seed extract, red clover, cat's claw, berberis root, and the ever popular echinacea and goldenseal. Many of the most helpful herbs are found in Rockland's main products: Liquid Logic and Liquid Life. Clark, to be mentioned later, also has many recommendations in this regard. Base your supplements on what problems you have, and whatever works for you-we are all different, and it is your responsibility to find out and speak up about what works for you specifically.

Silymarin, also known as milk thistle, contains some of the most potent liver protecting substances known. Many might think helping their livers out is not necessary as they lead healthy lives overall, but they might be surprised by how much damage the liver is sustaining from this toxic world in the meantime. And for those who ever took drugs, prescription or otherwise, or eaten many unnatural foods, or have had to deal with metal toxicity, or many other woes, liver protection and assistance is urgently recommended. Moonlight health offers an excellent liver support formula in this regard.

Cayenne is an herb that deserves special mention. As a fellow at this link argues, cayenne should always be included in any herbal collection, since it will make the other herbs work better: http://www.healingdaily.com/detoxification-diet/cayenne.htm . Its primary ingredient, capsaicin, may well be one of the most powerful circulatory stimulants known. The article linked here discourages capsule consumption in this case, saying the brain should be in on the loop of digestion from the tongue onward for full benefit. Some who cannot handle cayenne pepper directly may wish to disperse it liberally in drinks, like tomato juice. More on cayenne below.

Is that not a *lot* of supplements? Maybe, but *none of them are necessary if you just eat food the way it is grown naturally.* The better you eat, the less supplements you need.

It's your call.

When all is said and done, it is debatable whether a single extraordinary method mentioned in this whole book would be advisable at all if your diet was flawless. According to Dr. Howell, wild animals have no diseases—and they eat only raw foods. They only seem to get diseased when living close to man. And as far as the wisdom of the native American Indian medicine men goes, the Eskimos seem to have done them one better—they not only had no medicine men, but had no need of any—they, too, ate only raw foods.

3. Detox

If you do not eat well and refuse to supplement, you may find yourself toxic. In rare cases, those who eat right can become toxic from environmental contaminants. Such toxicity must then be rectified by the organs of detoxification in the body.

The body has six main paths of detoxification: the bowel, the liver, the kidneys, the skin, the lymphatic system, and the lungs, and all of these can become glutted with pollution.

So is there a simple and easy way to clean these pathways all at once if we are seriously ill? Well, an idea from antiquity can certainly be used with as much ease today as it was then: the fast. There are many different kinds of fasts, each with its associated advantages and drawbacks, but Stanley Burroughs believes that the fast he describes is, as he calls it, *The Master Cleanser* (fax # 1-775-972-4899 to request more info, and the booklet is sometimes still available in health food stores). So what does the master cleanser involve? It includes 1) A laxative herb tea, taken first thing in the morning and lastly at night to loosen up toxins in the intestine, with the possible substitution of a drink made of 1 quart warm water with 2 level teaspoons of sea salt taken on an empty stomach in the morning replacing the morning herb tea and 2) as many of the special cleanse drinks as desired per day, with an average of 5 to 10 taken by most people. The special drinks include 10 oz medium hot purified or spring water, two tablespoons organic lemon juice freshly squeezed, two tablespoons all natural maple syrup (lighter amounts to lose weight, heavier to gain) and 1/10 teaspoon cayenne pepper. Note that some may profit from heating the salt water drink up a bit before taking it while the contents are warm. The fast can last 10 days, or up to 40 in the case of serious illness.

Special precautions must be taken in coming off the diet, and these should not be ignored. Further details are of course in the booklet called *The Master Cleanser,* and more details are also publicly available at the most wondrous website curezone.com, which has a great overview of many health subjects presented here. *This fast, especially combined with exercise, may be the most surefire way of losing weight known.* To lose weight one simply must burn more calories than are consumed. Mineral supplements can aid in this task, as can pyruvate consumption according to Dr. Wallach. Another outstandingly simple way to accomplish weight loss is by using digestive enzymes. Just set a weight loss rate of however many pounds per week you wish to lose (without being absurd), then experiment with enzyme doses both at meals *and* between meals until you find the dose that accomplishes your goal. You may find yourself frequenting the toilet, flushing the pounds away, so do not be surprised if enzyme consumption has this result—it simply means the enzymes are doing exactly what they are supposed to do.

The fast is a method of cleansing all organs at once and assisting the body to solve virtually *any* major health crisis, but getting out certain pollutants in the body is another major aspect of detox, and other tools can greatly assist in this regard. Though when most people think of illness, they usually think about pathogens: parasites like tiny worms, bacteria like staphylococcus, and viruses like adenovirus, pathogens are usually only half of the picture one can find in an unhealthy body-contamination being the other. Indeed, the two often go hand in hand.

Some of the contaminants are solvents. Solvents are simply liquids in which other substances are dissolved. In modern society, there are a great many manufacturing processes in which one substance is dissolved in another, but the solvent will survive the processing of a product in such a way as to get inside our bodies after we unwrap the product from the grocery store, even if the solvent is not mentioned on the list of ingredients. Among the more dangerous solvents are benzene, wood alcohol/methanol, propyl alcohol, xylene, toluene, methyl ethyl ketone, and methyl butyl ketone.

The good news is that these solvents are easily gotten rid of. Simply stop consuming the products that contain them! How can you do this? A technical way would be to get or build a Clark syncrometer (described below) and test your products, and use only the ones your own tests show to be safe. But an even cheaper way is to simply not put things inside your body made in a factory-go natural!

These solvents can damage organs. A typical disease cycle might run like this: A person eats manufactured food. The body has trouble digesting it, so it ends up as impacted black waste in the intestine. Parasites, bacteria and viruses arrive on their daily rounds and are delighted that a mansion has been built for them, and they promptly take up residence in the intestine. When the intestine gets backed up, these parasites are escorted via limo to the bloodstream, where they go hunting for summer homes. In a normal healthy person, they are out of luck, as the immune defense system will kill them where they stand, but today the parasites are thrilled to find a person who is consuming lovely beers and soft drinks and bottled waters which may be contaminated with wood alcohol, propyl alcohol and/or benzene. Among the damaged organs are the lungs, the pancreas and the liver. Some parasites decide to colonize each organ. The result is a fellow with asthma, diabetes, and liver malfunction.

Again, to prevent this, try to work with stuff as close to the way it occurs in nature and avoid even small amounts of solvent contamination. Solvents will generally exit your system in a week provided you do not replenish their reserves.

It is intriguing that after all of the technical science presented by Dr. Clark in her books on curing all diseases, the principal conclusion she draws is two simple words: go primitive.

Another form of contamination is heavy metal toxicity. Heavy metals can be absorbed from a poor water supply system, where copper, lead and other metals leak from joints or pipes. Although the body does need minerals like these, it needs them in a useable, or bioavailable form, and the big nasty clumps in water are too much to handle. They can however, eventually pollute the body and be exploited by bacterial invaders. For example, some bacteria thrive on nickel. While drinking water may be a serious source of metal toxicity, probably the worst offender by far is dental fillings. Commonly metal dental fillings are called silver, but such fillings may be 50% or more mercury, a deadly poison to our system. Dr Clark is quite vocal about the importance of getting this metal out of our mouths as fast as we can. There is a great deal of evidence suggesting that metal toxicity is a necessary precondition for certain parasitic infections, leading to major diseases like Alzheimer's and Parkinson's. What kind of evidence? Well, would you believe there have been cases of Alzheimer's symptoms radically reducing within days of people having their metal fillings removed, sometimes within hours? Such cases are on record. Please see *Suppressed Inventions* or *The Key To Ultimate Health* for more.

So what can we do about tooth metal? One option strongly recommended by Dr Clark is to have the metal removed and the fillings replaced with composite. This may be costly, but can be far less costly than drug lord alternatives offered to one facing serious disease. It should be noted that most composites are only less toxic than metal, and not perfect solutions to this problem. In *The Key To Ultimate Health,* lasers are used to solve various dental problems, but this can be a costly process.

Another option to remove metals lurking in the body is a process called chelation. Chelation is a word that comes from root words that translate as "to claw". Chelation is a process whereby annoying things in us are clawed out by chemicals (typically amino acids, proteins or enzymes) that are ideal for binding with bad guys and sending them to the excretory system for prompt garbage encounters.

Two simple chelators available in health food stores are histidine and thioctic acid (also called alpha lipoic acid). If you know someone with Alzheimer's or Parkinson's, it could not hurt to at least give chelation a try and see if there are improvements. Garlic can chelate cadmium, lead and mercury. A more intense form of chelation therapy is offered at previously mentioned moonlight health.com. For about $80, one can order products in tablet form called Longevity Plus 2 and Oral Chelation 2. In clinical lab tests, the elimination rates of metals from the body were as follows: for 14 patients, the average % increase in

excretion after just one day: Aluminum: 229% Arsenic: 661 %
Cadmium 276% Lead 350% Mercury 773% Nickel 9,439%
These results speak for themselves. Fasting does not
seem to have the ability to withdraw heavy metals as well as
chelation. Reportedly the most powerful form of chelation is
EDTA chelation, available from vrp.com (by the way--want to
protect yourself from nuclear radiation? Potassium iodate can help,
available from vrp.com, (along with xylitol products)). EDTA is
also available in Rockland's premier cost effective chelation
product, Cardio EZ. Liver and kidney support herbs, like those
available from moonlight health, can help chelation efforts.

The possibilities for teeth shine from a startling
footnote from history where those who ate flawlessly with proper
nutrition as described here (some have stressed additionally that
supplementing with Calcium, Magnesium and Boron aids this
effort, as found in yet another Rockland formulation), and/or in
pursuing the health methods of Dr. Ray, whom we shall return to
shortly, supposedly regenerated their teeth with such force that
their metal fillings were eventually ejected. *It would appear that
only the nutrition program presented in this book has led to such
instances of body regeneration—a most compelling argument for
its power.* The new regeneration formula at the back of the book is
now being investigated for its ability to accomplish teeth
regeneration. Results will be announced in future printings.

Because of the dangers of metal contamination,
perhaps one might give thought to the constant use of metal in our
daily lives. We have metal cookware, silverware and buildings,
and sometimes consume quantities of aluminum from deodorant
and soft drink cans, while many will go so far as not only to place
metal in contact with their earlobes, but pierce their bodies all over
with metal. The health consequences of such metal toxicity shall
undoubtedly lead to many a grim reckoning. It is also interesting to
note that there are likely many who have commented on what
ingenious innovations metal skyscrapers are, but I wonder if the
ancients would have been impressed-metals can be toxic to us,
while many of the ancient stones might actually have had minerals

in them that would have benefitted us from our contact with them more than harmed us.

In any case, you now have another tool available to you in natural healing.

The fast, and chelation attempt to remove trouble from the entire body at once, but the less ambitious may wish to pursue revitalizing one detox pathway at a time. If you do so, understand that of all the pathways, the bowel, as Dr Jensen states, is king of them all.

As reported by Dr. Jensen, in his book, *Dr. Jensen's Guide To Better Bowel Care,* there are a great many health conditions and diseases that are promptly eliminated with a newly cleansed bowel. Two other doctors independently reached the same conclusion about the bowel. Asthma apparently was one problem that could never last if the bowel were cleaned. Decades ago, many surgeons noted that a number of other conditions in their patients besides their primary trouble improved drastically when parts of the colon were removed. The same effect from colon surgery can be accomplished in several less costly ways. One way is to use the colon cleaning procedure described in Jensen's book. Another way is to use a Colon Cleanse available at health food stores such as Wild Oats and others. For the cost of about 10 to 15 bucks, a one month colon cleanse can rid the intestines of impacted, black, foul smelling waste (graphically illustrated in Jensen's book and not for the faint of heart) that not only prevents the proper absorption of key nutrients, but also acts as an ideal breeding ground for a great many pathogens: parasites, bacteria, and viruses. Remove their home base, and you will have a much easier time dealing with the escapees from home base in your other organs.

A one month cleanse is usually not recommended for four consecutive weeks, but rather for a two week starting phase, followed by a three week interlude, then concluded with another two week finishing phase. Be sure to remain well hydrated, and further remember that flaxseed oil supplementation can be an additional aid in keeping things moving along smoothly. Bentonite clay, also available in health food stores, may be added to a bowel cleanse program for even better results. This clay has been used for centuries by many native peoples. The negative ions in the clay are ideal for binding to the commonly large, positively charged clogging clumps caught in our systems. The clay may also be used to clean and revitalize the skin, and draw out the toxins lurking in cysts. As one enthusiastic champion of the clay approach to life has stated, "I have been eating dirt for years, and I love it." Believe it or not, there is a book entitled *The Clay Cure* devoted exclusively to this topic.

The Rockland Corporation, once again with cost effective wholesale rates, offers a cleanse that includes bentonite clay for less than nine dollars. Brenda Watson offers still another cleanse called Cleanse Smart from Renewlife, that offers backup herbal support for the liver and kidneys and overall system which may suffer from nasty spillover during the cleanse process. Burroughs, mentioned before, recommends a laxative herbal tea morning and night, with a salt water drink possibly substituting for the morning drink. Whatever method you choose, find out if the method cleanses the *whole* tract, as many methods like colonics often clean only a small part. The salt water cleanse is cheap and very effective in this regard. Note that one salt water drink will not cleanse the whole tract—it may take several drinks over weeks to regain cleanliness—the goal, again, is bowel movements in true proportion to meals.

One should also note that the same things which recur again and again as villains to avoid--coffee, tea, tobacco, alcohol and high protein foods to name a few again-- also just so happen to be highly damaging to the intestinal microorganisms. Hurting them is worse than shooting yourself in the foot, because your entire body will suffer once those hardworking helpful colonies are wrecked. Restoring their levels might begin with something as simple as yogurt consumption, but one can also find formulations with major gut helpers like lactobacillus, acidophilus, chlorella (fantastic at promoting the binding of certain toxins) and spirulina, so look around. Be aware that drug lords love to use antibiotics—a solution about as graceful and elegant as using a nuclear bomb for rapid city street cleaning—please try to be smarter than this, as the good microorganisms as well as the bad are indiscriminately slaughtered by this witless action. Many factors influence whether supplemented microorganisms thrive or perish. Even some of the health methods in this book can harm good microorganisms, so never forget the goal is to use restorative methods only when health is compromised, and then perform maintenance sparingly as needed.

PH, the degree of acidity or alkalinity, has a big effect on bacterial fates. If you read the article below on colloidal silver you can get a succinct account of the importance of pH. At Rockland you can get 15 feet of pH paper for about 5 bucks to check yourself. Coral calcium (at least, that not contaminated with lead, mercury, or cesium) (that sold by Rockland is supposedly such a one) can be an elaborate way to restore normal pH for those who refuse to use nature's completely free, ultimate pH normalizer—water. Rockland minerals and ingested minerals in general stabilize pH, and create a joyful, strong, teeming intestinal community.

Yet another insight which can jar one into appreciating the majesty of the bowel comes from a case reported in England of a man supposedly living to be 160 years old (he reportedly had a 120+ year child to prove it). The peculiarity led to an autopsy to determine the reason for longevity. The only oddity found was a perfectly shaped bowel—which rarely happens anywhere. Most bowels are misshapen from poor eating habits.

Since the bowel is indeed of such prime importance, it would be worthwhile to slam a few points home while on the subject. When food is undigested, it decays: proteins rot, carbohydrates ferment, and fats go rancid. Such a mess becomes the ideal breeding ground for parasites, bacteria and viruses of *any* negative species. There seems to be a counterproductive monomania when people think of curing disease, when individuals think that the crime will soon be solved once one villainous bacterium is named, but this approach usually fails. One villain is named and eradicated, yet the problem persists. Dr. Clark tells us that viruses may piggy back on bacteria, and bacteria on parasites. And in many people who have created toxic bowels, they may have *several* species of invaders bent on attack. *Thus your best strategy remains to wipe out* **all** *the villains.* It does not matter if the villains eventually set up a colony in the pancreas, lungs, or liver, or wherever—*the bowel is almost always home base,* and the bad guys really have no prayer of staying inside you if a quick bowel transit time is strictly kept, and pathogen reserves are never reinforced. *It does not matter what the name of the disease is, how many syllables it has, how new or exotic it is: if you keep the bowel (and the mouth) clean, and the bad guys have no home base— THAT IS MOST OF THE BATTLE!!!*

As for the undigested matter, note that undigested fats can clog and clump red blood cells, warping their shape, and damaging their ability to distribute vital, lifegiving, immune system energizing oxygen. Thus it is especially important to cleanse the liver, to ensure proper fat digestion.

The liver can be cleaned by the use of a liver cleanse procedure, described in the frontier crossing book *The Cure For All Diseases* by naturopathic Doctor Hulda Clark, and also described for free on the web: http://www.kidneycleanse.com/. One can also go to the Clark website at drclark.net for more info. Liver function can be impaired by accumulated stones, often formed around an invader the body could not otherwise deal with, but these stones may be stuck in the gall bladder or liver ducts and require some assistance in disposal. Such blockage can lead to pain in various regions of the body, especially the back. Dr. Clark further insists that allergies will weaken and eventually disappear entirely if liver cleanses are used regularly—twice a year for maintenance, but once every two weeks if necessary. The liver cleanse procedure has been safely used in thousands of cases, and involves the drinking of epsom salts and water at specific intervals, to be followed before bedtime with a drink of olive oil and fresh pink grapefruit juice. The following morning more epsom salts are consumed, and the stones pass by easily through the intestines. Some may wish to consume extra water to offset the lost water from the cleanse. Unhealthy people tend to pass stones that are brown, whereas healthier people pass stones that are green, the color of healthy bile, a key liver fluid. In one case, a man whose eyes showed a yellowish cast, from the pigment bilirubin that expresses liver distress, passed a thousand tiny stones and the yellow cast soon disappeared from his eyes. Another woman easily avoided costly gall bladder surgery. Please follow each and every rule as described freely in the Clark books and website before following this procedure. Also be aware that the rich drug companies, sensing a dire threat to their profits, have launched a smear campaign against Dr Clark. Please evaluate all arguments about what is really going in the health marketplace, such as those presented in the fantastic book *Suppressed Inventions And Other Discoveries* by Jonathan Eisen, before turning away from field tested nature and going back on briefly tested drugs.

Since the liver is involved in the production of cholesterol, some misconceptions on that subject should be clarified.

At the present time, with heart disease running so high, many of you may be more eager to figure out how to get fatty cholesterol removed from the blood as opposed to heavy metals, and will you not be surprised to learn that all of this fuss about cholesterol is nothing but nonsense, an utter farce and inane hoax?

The first clue any amateur scientist should have wondered about was why, if cholesterol was so bad, does the liver daily churn out vast quantities of the stuff? Rather strange of the liver to kill us that way, would you not think? The next clue would come on the day in physiology class when your teacher draws out for you the chemical structures of all those hormones sex crazed humans get so uppity about. For what do we see plain as day on the chalkboard? That they are built from (drum roll) cholesterol (good to go with the rim shot)!

Further, cholesterol is essential in the construction of cells. Dr. Wallach says that the myelin sheath insulation of almighty brain cells is pretty much 100% cholesterol, so does eliminating cholesterol really sound smart? If so, maybe you need some cholesterol! He goes on to say if your doctors recommend lowering your cholesterol below 200, flee from them because they'll kill you. He considers blood cholesterol levels of 200 to 275 normal, and believes they should not be lowered further should one find their cholesterol at this level. Still not had enough?

Yet another clue that cholesterol is not the bogeyman comes from stacks of evidence concerning earlier generations of Americans who gulped down milk and cream and butter like they had bells around their necks yet still had nowhere near the levels of heart disease today. See the book from Dr. Donsbach on heart disease available from Rockland for a most telling history of this subject.

In a similar spirit, a fellow in the United Kingdom once prescribed higher levels of milk, butter and cream to the population and found disease rates dropping quickly. So if cholesterol is so useful, why on earth are authorities trying desperately to convince us otherwise? If you guessed the reason has something to do with money, consider yourself a genius and give yourself a free carrot. The money was to be made by-take a guess anyone? The margarine folks, among others!

So how exactly did they sneak that cholesterol link to heart disease in and get so many to swallow it? Let us go over a little history.

I suppose if one were feeling egregiously generous, you could grant that there MIGHT have been a vaguely reasonable origin to the idea that cholesterol was a villain. As recounted in the history supplied by Barry Groves (please see http://www.secondopinions.co.uk/cvd_index.htm for more) a number of servicemen were found with bad hearts and cholesterol clumps at the site of damage. But as any wise bystander can see, you cannot accuse cholesterol merely for the record of being at the scene of the crime. With that mentality one might wish to arrest all those suspicious paramedics that always seem to be on the spot at accidents. Another problem with yelling at cholesterol for its location is that, cholesterol being so essential to our functioning, it pretty much belongs, well, everywhere in the body. Another problem with making cholesterol a public enemy is that it is often found mixed with other nasty things at the sites of damage, and these other things may be more to blame for any troubles. This much ballyhooed distinction between high density lipoprotein or HDL and low density lipoprotein, or LDL is really not much to toot a horn about either. Uffe Ravnskov, (consult his works or http://www.ravnskov.nu/cholesterol.htm for more), explains that HDL helps cholesterol get from the liver to our organs, and LDL helps it get from the organs to our liver. So why is one good and one bad? Well, asking the bad guys to explain themselves is always frustrating, because when they talk they kind of look like drunken men scrambling through obstacle courses. Ravnskov tries to explain this odd position in his material, but there is no reason to bother giving this silliness any more press time here. If any do hear an explanation, you may wish to tape it and play it back to any who require a sleep aid.

But what about the main idea so often heard in the news, about clogging fat in the blood? How does that really work? Well, here is really what happens, so strap yourself in for the little rollercoaster ride.

When people do not eat natural foods, whether fatty or not, the liver may become impaired with stones, which usually encase microbe invaders. Too many stones lead to less bile production. Less bile means less fat digestion, and this fat coats the intestinal walls. Now stop the film and watch to see who is entering the left side of the frame at this point. What type of fat is the kind most likely not to be digested? Cholesterol from butter? Heck, no. As partially mentioned before, the real criminals here are actually hydrogenated oils, trans fatty acids and other bizarre fatty acid forms like those in margarine. Just because some fat is not being digested does not mean you can call it all cholesterol and blame dairy. OK, now we can roll film again. The blood vessels then pull this fat into the bloodstream, when they were really hoping to grab some better nutrients. The blood cells get coated with this fat and cannot deliver oxygen to cells. What is worse is that these fatty cells may bind to calcium, leading to plaques and atherosclerosis and vessel clogging. The combination with calcium is another mighty interesting part. Why would people have too much calcium floating around? The answer is that too many phosphates in the diet such as those from soft drinks (and meats, again we were meant to be herbivores) cause the body to release calcium from bones to deal with the excess phosphates. Is it possible that the soda and meat folks are engaged along with others in a costly game of point the finger at the dairy folks? But I suppose "Have a cola and no bile" is not quite as catchy for an ad campaign.

DA Lopez says sometimes cholesterol with pointy crystals on it is seen as causing damage, but cholesterol does not typically have pointy crystals on it, so the normal routine has obviously been broken in some way. We already know that calcium and phosphates can form crystals, so some suspects do emerge.

What is even more ludicrous is when people try to solve this apparent "problem" by encouraging the elimination of fat from the diet. This actually causes the liver to desperately crank *up* cholesterol levels to get needed fats into circulation, leading to liver overdrive, and the whole mess gets worse. As we stated before, fat itself is not harmful, what is harmful is an imbalanced intake of fat. That was the story we gave you at the beginning, and we are stickin' to it. In addition to the aforementioned Ravnskov info, you may wish to read the writings of Sally Fallon, and Mary Enig. Search for their work on the web and the previously mentioned website.

As has been stated by many an inside scientist, serum or blood cholesterol is not in direct proportion to dietary cholesterol. Since the liver daily churns out its own supply, it is only logical that this be the case. Whatever way we look at it naturally, cholesterol cannot be blamed for heart disease. So once again, we see the moneygrubbers trying to tell us nature is screwy, when it is actually their profit margins that are screwy. One would tell those folks nice try, but frankly after a while they just seem wacky.

The liver cleanse is powerful in expelling gallstones, whether hard or soft, and improving fat digestion, but if you expect to get the full benefits of raw foods with the greatest speed after living a toxic life, then recharge your liver with liver herbs. Moonlight health offers a great liver herb combination in its liver support product, designed to help revitalize livers damaged from toxic environments, addictions, drugs whether medical or recreational, or just life on this polluted planet. Dr. Clark, in the aforementioned book, lists many herbs that can be taken in combination to enhance liver function. Of course, the classic liver protector herb is silymarin, also known as milk thistle, available cheaply with tumeric from Rockland. The coffee enemas described below also greatly aid the liver and sweep many toxins away from the body.

The liver filters the blood, and it can do a better job when the blood flow itself optimal. How do you optimize blood flow? Try cayenne pepper!

See this link for more:
http://www.healingdaily.com/detoxification-diet/cayenne.htm

Understand that no part of your body can feel pain if it has optimal blood flow, which brings in vital nutrients, water and oxygen, and removes toxic waste and leftovers from cellular metabolism. Got chronic pain? Make your blood move with cayenne!!

Blood *pressure* is, of course, the province of the kidneys, and hence we arrive at our next detox pathway. The kidneys are generally easy to maintain, provided one follows the above rules and avoids those foods that can damage the kidneys over time. Popular teas (especially iced tea) and even hot cocoa can lead to oxalate crystal formations, one of the seven types of kidney stones described in Clark's book. Soft drinks are especially damaging. They contain high amounts of phosphates, which can form crystals that impair kidney function (not to mention that phosphates leach calcium from the bones and weaken them). They also contain damaging sweeteners (see article at Nexus archive: http://www.nexusmagazine.com/SugarBlues.html) and an acidic pH that upsets the natural body balance. One could call them liquid poison and not be far off, so help the kidneys and avoid them. Be sure to get calcium and phosphorus in more useable forms (like the Rockland minerals) and the crystals will go away. Uric acid crystals are the consequence of undigested protein—and since you already know now that protein digesting enzymes break down undigested protein, stick with your enzymes!

The Amazon Herb Company at amazonherb.net offers many herbs straight from the rainforest that can aid not only in kidney support but other areas as well, such as colon cleansing. The company is working with native people to save the rainforests by working with nature, rather than levelling it as so many wish to do. Bear in mind that, for many of those natives, the diseases of our world are unknown, and their leading causes of deaths are snake bites and trees falling unexpectedly.

Blood pressure is most often adversely affected more by caffeine intake than any other factor, including salt, though putting refined salt on everything is definitely wrong, especially the common sodium chloride variety. Consider the ideas of Dr Clark on the use of sea salt. Also consider the ideas presented at curezone.com regarding what is called the salt cure. Unrefined salt contains many vital trace minerals that, it would appear, have been part of animal history for millions of years, and which have only recently been banished in the last 150 years or so by moneyloving industry. Still, since Eskimos eating raw foods without any additional salt whatsoever maintain optimal chloride levels, salt should be considered a remedial measure for those eating too many processed foods more than a natural requirement.

But again, hydrate yourself well with clean water and healthy juices, get fiber from sources like whole grain breads and vegetables, eat the right fats, supplement with minerals, and kiss high blood pressure goodbye. Any further assistance you might need you can get from any one of the pioneers on this book. Everyone here can beat high blood pressure with one ankle tied to their left elbow. Nature-for lack of a better word-is good. Nature works. Michael Douglas may soon have a movie on this, too.

Your heart rate should ideally be close to 85 beats per minute-if yours is too high you may want to cut down on beverages that hurt the kidneys and try drinking better fluids. In addition to downing 100% natural organic fruit juices, the consumption of fresh watermelon can also be a fantastic aid for the kidneys. Some have dissolved stones with high watermelon intake.

The aforementioned Carlson Wade, in his booklet called *Juice Power*, tosses in that the juices of cantaloupe, nectarines, peaches and papaya are also great for the kidneys.

So now you can add methods to eradicate heart disease, America's number one killer, and several to beat high blood pressure, to your little bag o tricks.

Clean water is a great aid to health in general, yet most city tap water is impure. And Dr. Clark, mentioned earlier, claims that most bottled waters are contaminated with solvents which can be even more damaging to the body. You may wish to invest in a water filter such as those offered by the Rockland Corporation, the lifetime 480 being an example. This 60 odd dollar filter can almost completely remove sediment, the chlorine and chlorine compounds that can damage the body (leaving water out for a few hours also releases the chlorine), trihalomethanes, dangerous heavy metals such as lead, copper, and more, as well as hazardous fluoride. For more web info, see the website reachforlife.com, or call 1-800-258-5028. Dr. Clark (see more below) has now thrown her hat into the water filter ring—see her site for more. There are also units called Grander units, based on the work of the laudable Viktor Schauberger. These supposedly vitalize water to an otherwise highly unlikely ideal state—but they can be expensive. An interesting note from these units highlights the significance of clean water. Experiments showed that bathwater in a typical situation became cleaner after people bathed in it—in other words, more dirt went into them when bathing than came out. Water treated by a Grander unit had the opposite result. Strange to think how bathing might be making many people unclean… A goal that all can test for is the presence of low surface tension in water, which can be studied in capillary tubes. The lower the surface tension, the less it will rise in a capillary tube, and the better the water, Magnets, ozone generators, or the item of your choice could lower the surface tension of your water, making it—and you—healthier. Even so small a step as to purchase some tap water conditioner from pet stores may make a difference in the struggle for optimum health. Another superior water company offering bottled water can be found in oxywater, website at oxywater.com, phone number 1-877-699-9287. You can also call 1-888-877-2322 and speak with distributor James Johnson for arrangements. This superior water is spreading currently into many retail chains, so check around. Some other companies are offering alkalized water to help push pH in a helpful direction.

Many cities fluoridate water. Though the public in general is unaware of the dangers, fluoride is well known to be an extremely harmful substance by many scientists. For more on the dangers of fluoride, see *Suppressed Inventions and Other Discoveries*, and on the web read the sworn affidavit of doctor A K Susheela, a PhD for those of you that means something to, who worked directly with fluoride effects for years (link: http://www.rvi.net/-fluoride/susheela.htm). Fluoride should not be in toothpaste, as it does nothing to help teeth, but can definitely harm them. Perhaps the best toothpaste would be an old recipe the previous generations have long known and trusted: a little bit of baking soda with clean water. Dr Katz at www.therabreath.com has additional dental care recommendations. One may rinse afterwards with food grade hydrogen peroxide, a substance we shall return to shortly, and enjoy great teeth for a lifetime, all other factors being equal, though Clark does not recommend peroxide rinsing for those with metal fillings, as the peroxide may react with the metal. Rockland offers a Superoxy mouth wash.

Other home hygiene products besides fluoride toothpaste can also hurt the body. Dr. Clark goes into great detail on such matters in her book. In each case, whether it be soap, shampoo, deodorant or toothpaste, many home hygiene products sold in stores are not very safe, and cheaper, more healthy alternatives are readily available. One company offers some alternatives at realpurity.com, and another at aubreyorganics.com. One may also order products from Dr. Clark, or use the ideas she presents to make your own. Another website for the do it yourselfer is makestuff.com. Remember, in today's less than pristine world, the body needs all the help it can get to maintain cleanliness, both internal and external.

The next organ of detox is the skin, the largest organ in the body. Keep the skin glowing by use of a skin brush, available in stores like Wild Oats and The Body Shop. Apply seven strokes to each body part, each stroke directed towards the heart where appropriate. Many, though, recommend not brushing sensitive areas like the breast, genitals, neck and face. One woman stopped using moisturizers after getting accustomed to this procedure, as her old skin sloughed off and the new skin came in fresh and vibrant. Always brush the skin when dry, and do not overdo the brushing—constipation may result! In other words, so many toxins may exit the skin the intestines may be left with little to do. Another woman whose ovarian cancer was cured in 7 weeks had hydrogen peroxide baths preceded by skin brushing as part of her regimen.

Another way to enhance the skin is to treat it well nutritionally. Soap can dry the skin and rob it of moisture. While most bathe in less than ideal water, some steps to help the skin retain moisture may be recommended. One such recommendation would be to explore the possibilities of treating the skin with coconut oil. The aforementioned author Fife has a whole chapter devoted to the benefits of applying coconut oil to the skin. It becomes visibly healthier, and this also applies to the hair. One can take a tiny amount of oil, place it in a tiny amount of water in a pot on the stove, mildly heat the mix briefly, dunk a comb in it, comb the hair till the hair is damp, let sit an hour, then rinse in the shower. You will feel the difference.

Coconut oil can help rejuvenate the skin, but skin regeneration is tackled in a later chapter.

After the skin comes the lymphatic system, a vitally crucial general body plumbing purification system. The lymphatic system works by a pumping action, and the primary nodes, or pump zones, are located in areas where your body moves a great deal, such as near the armpits. Therefore the easiest way to get the lymph to flow is to exercise, plain and simple. The lymphatic system, in some extreme cases, may be so overburdened that exercise may not be enough. The brilliant health pioneer, Gaston Naessens, website at cerbe.com, and whose story is also featured in *Suppressed Inventions*, has developed a product called 714 x to directly assist a troubled lymphatic system. He has eliminated cancer with this method. For those of you who will complain that you are being given too many ways to destroy cancer, apologies are offered. One may spend as much as $500 to get his products and understand how to use them, but when a man can keep cancer at bay far more cheaply than the typical drug approaches in which thousands upon thousands of dollars are spent on ineffective drugs, one may wish to consider the Naessens research first. Another method of cleaning the lymph is mentioned rather pointedly by Dr. Samuel West. He calls the method lymphasizing, but all that really means is jumping on a minitrampoline. For those too ill to stand on one, you can sit and bounce. Even a few bounces can help. West reports that some severely ill people kicked loose so many toxins from a few bounces they could actually do no more. As with all things, go at your own pace. West definitely views clean lymph as a matter of life or death—review his research to understand more!

It should be stressed at this point that there is a difference between loosening and binding systemic toxins and removing them from the body completely. Enzymes are better at the former task, but rely on the bowels or other detox pathways to finish the job—which they may or may not be able to do. Chelators also grab toxins as the enzymes do, but also rely on the detox pathways to finish the job. If all detox pathways are compromised, special methods may be necessary to insure the bound toxins are removed. According to the Gerson therapy, the coffee enema is wondrous on such an assignment, so see the Gerson therapy info presented earlier or this link for more: http://www.cleanse.net/coffee_enema.HTM. Again, cayenne, as described before, helps the circulatory system do its job. Oxygen therapies, explored next, are fantastic both in identifying and loosening toxins, and seeing to their removal.

As for the final organ of detox, the lungs, the cheapest way to maintain healthy lungs is simply to breathe correctly, drawing full breaths that work the diaphragm. Exercise, especially yoga, also helps to maintain lung health. Oxygen, in various forms such as peroxide, stabilized oxygen as sold in health food stores, and ozone generators, such as those sold at wateroz.com, can dramatically assist the lungs in getting back on track should they be at low power.

Asthmatics have abandoned their inhalers after working with oxygen therapies. A chronic emphysema patient was downgraded to basic emphysema after coughing up toxic globs expelled thanks to peroxide. Construction workers witnessed better breathing and lesser allergies.

In fact, oxygen is so flabbergasting in its power, it deserves its own special section.

4. Oxygen

Oxygen therapy is actually a realm unto itself. A researching pioneer by the name of Ed McCabe has written a most excellent book you may wish to investigate called *Oxygen Therapies,* and his new book *Flood Your Body With Oxygen* is also now available, and is a fountainhead of amazing information. Nathaniel Altman has written another useful book on the same topic called *Oxygen Healing Therapies.* Additionally relevant, Saul Pressman. has written a rather brilliant technical account you can read for free on the web entitled *The Story of Ozone* (link: http://www.ozonio.com.br/medical.htm). Oxygen destroys many harmful microbes, and oxygen in the form of hydrogen peroxide, h2o2, and ozone, o3, are especially potent.

Peroxide is cheap, costing about 15 bucks for a pint that may well last you a year or more. If you choose to explore peroxide, you will want to use FOOD GRADE hydrogen peroxide for oral applications. Drugstore brands have lower levels of purity, as they were not intended for oral use. Do you want to take a chance of burdening your body with an additional foreign substance when you are sick? Thought not. The percentage of food grade does not matter-there may exist 17%, 12%, whatever % (but note that dosages here are based on 35%--so if you get something half as strong, take twice as much, and so on). Reagent grade is also acceptable. Always take drops in distilled water, or other purified water, about 8 ounces worth. Take 1 drop day 1, 2 day 2, and so on until you find a personal maximum of drops you are comfortable and happy with-and NEVER OVERLOAD TO SOLVE A PROBLEM. MAX is 25 drops 3 times a day, though 10 at a time, *once* a day, should be plenty for most everyone once you have worked up to that level of drops. Men seem to tolerate it better than women. Some may wish to take this with juice (not carrot or banana—their oxygen enzymes will react too eagerly with the peroxide). DO NOT CONSUME PEROXIDE WITH MEALS-HAVE AT LEAST A HALF HOUR CUSHION ON BOTH SIDES, preferably much more, such as one hour clear before and two after. ONE MAN WHO BROKE THIS RULE SAW NO RESULTS FROM PEROXIDE. WHEN HE FOLLOWED THE RULES HE GOT BETTER IMMEDIATELY. DO NOT BREAK THE RULES!!!

Some may wish to enjoy a 3 week cleansing program (no, you do not have to take it for the rest of your life—again, you would not have to do much of anything extra if you eat right, exercise, and go unrefined), taking a drink a day until a personal max of drops is found, then holding that max until 3 weeks have gone by for general cleaning. One easy way to tell whether you might benefit from peroxide is to check the color of your blood the next opportunity that arises, perhaps during blood donation, or a checkup, or even an accidental cut. If your blood is a bright, beautiful red you are well oxygenated and may wish to forego oxygen therapy, if not, you may try to boost your oxygen levels, either with peroxide or the method of your choice.

PEROXIDE IS COMPLETELY NATURAL. Nature has known the power of peroxide for eons, even if man has not. Inside the cells of your body are organelles called peroxisomes--they contain natural hydrogen peroxide. If most people did not insist on eating such massive quantities of garbage and contaminating themselves with unnatural soaps, shampoos, metals, drinking water, deodorants and countless other things, the natural peroxide could keep up. As it is, it often gets overwhelmed, and this process of drinking peroxide can give your body a vital boost when your oxygen is low.

In some cases, the peroxide might trigger a battle in the body as the body gains the strength to fight off an attacker. Some people get rashes on occasion, others get boils (one woman wanted to try about 10 drops to start rather than starting slowly--her reward was a full body rash--FOLLOW THE RULES).

Rashes are NOT always bad things-they are merely your body's way of expelling intruders, as are boils. Healthy people often experience NO adverse effects of any kind. But one woman who was a smoker could not stand the sensation of peroxide in her system, it was like taking her back to the time before she puffed when cigarettes were repulsive--next trip to the doctor's he was amazed at how clean her blood had become--but such is the power of peroxide (you can expect cleaner blood to be found in all who have taken the peroxide to combat low oxygen). Another woman with root canals experienced sickness after taking the peroxide, and her gums hurt. She felt unhappy with the scuffle between peroxide and her gums, and felt this specific method was not for her in this case.

Root canals have been sharply criticized for the aftereffects dumped on the body, by Dr. Clark (to be explored further shortly), as well as by the Gersons, and for a more in depth treatment of dentistry, by all means consider the ideas of Richard Hansen in *The Key to Ultimate Health*. Dr. Clark has more thoughts on when peroxide might not be advisable, as does Ed McCabe. You have the option of contacting each with any questions you may have. You should understand that the peroxide will probably pick a fight with just about anything foreign in your body, so take this into account and make your choices accordingly. Decide for yourself what your circumstances, your strength and endurance are before moving forward. In any event, as with all methods on this book, if you feel certain that something is not working quite right, or you are uncomfortable with a procedure, by all means stop what you are doing immediately and please do more research with the materials offered here—that is what they are there for.

Those who find oral peroxide "too weird" may wish to try an alternative form of oxygen, called stabilized oxygen. Actually, McCabe does not recommend food grade peroxide for oral use any longer, believing other products deliver oxygen more effectively. Again, ask the health food stores if they have STABILIZED OXYGEN, then follow the instructions on the package, and use in the same way as peroxide. Tobinfarms.com also offers additional powerful oxygen products, like the impressive Hydroxygen Plus and Oxygen Boost. Rockland, as usual awake on the health front, offers its own stabilized oxygen product, Oxy-Gen, giving the same effect as food grade peroxide, but a tad tastier. For research, again, read the excellent books *Oxygen Therapies* and *Flood Your Body With Oxygen* by Ed McCabe, (website at edmccabe.org or misteroxygen.com) who will tell you of how oxygen (in peroxide form, among other forms) can fight acne, asthma, allergies, arthritis, candida, and countless other diseases, including cancer and AIDS (note that in more extreme cases you will need to seek a qualified doctor to administer the peroxide intravenously). Otto Warburg, a Nobel Prize winner (for those of you to whom that means something) insists that cancer cannot persist in the presence of oxygen. Countless case histories support this claim. You may also wish to check out the work of Kurt Donsbach and others in this regard at oxytherapy.com See also oxytherapies.com for more of the same.

Allergies, to the more alert researcher, sound silly as they are currently defined—as the body's completely inappropriate reaction to a nontoxic substance. Nature is repeatedly slandered by the ignorant and later exonerated by the wise. Dr. Clark claims that in the case of a wheat allergy, the individual is likely full of parasites and Kojic acid, for example--remove the garbage, no "allergy". She also says that some who claim to be allergic to milk are actually reacting to *salmonella* or *shigella*, and the lack of enzymes in the pasteurized milk—clean the milk, restore the enzymes, no allergy. People claim to be allergic to animals like cats and dogs, but these, according to Dr. Clark, often donate their parasites to us—so if we later have a reaction to the animal, is it the animal or its parasites that are most to blame? Would anyone ever be allergic to a cat or dog free of parasites and toxins?

Would anyone be allergic to anything if they themselves had a clean bowel, clean liver, ample enzymes, and richly oxygenated blood? It would seem there is no such case on record.

Use the methods described here and see. Is it possible that the term "allergies" is a term we throw at our ignorance of the consequences of having parasites and the principles of healthful living?

For oxygen skeptics, try this simple test in using the power of oxygen: buy some apple cider, then place maybe 5-10 drops of 35% food grade peroxide in it. The cider will convert back to fresh apple juice with a change in color! In other words, microbes just got wiped out. Also, you will find that milk can be preserved far longer with peroxide (possibly indefinitely). If pasteurization is so great, why does milk go bad so fast after a week? Try the peroxide and taste (or smell) the graphic difference in milk at two weeks. (Note: the instructions not to mix peroxide with food are for when you are using the peroxide for YOUR health--but of course it is ok to help preserve food with it.) You can also clean food with peroxide. Simply reduce down the 35% to a 3% solution in distilled water, and place in a squirt/spray bottle. Spray your fresh produce with 3%. Also spray the 3% solution on any rashes or skin infections or bruises. In one case, a woman had a cast on too tight. When it was removed, the skin was purple and black and she could not move her hand. After treatment with 3% peroxide solution, the hand returned to normal. In another case, a woman had menstrual pains all her life, and has only recently found some peace from oral peroxide. In still another case, a man suffering from a lethal fungal infection went to about 10 doctors, including ones at the Mayo clinic, and not only were they unskilled enough to diagnose his condition, but once the condition was known to them they were helpless to stop it. The man took intravenous peroxide and noticed an immediate improvement, with a bonus that his old gout markings also promptly disappeared. Later when he used ozone insufflation he became even better. When he cleaned his colon he was almost back to top form, and continues his amazing recovery. Another woman using ozone insufflation to combat cancer was shocked to see about forty feet of impacted waste exit from her colon—and quite content when her cancer marker plummeted to nothing thereafter.

Also note that one can bathe in peroxide, putting about one cup of 35% into a half tub, two for a full one, or more next time if you are comfy, making sure not to let the 35% hit your skin undiluted by more water. While we are mentioning water so often, we can mention that the separate authors Donsbach and Bhatmanghelidj have small books covering the topic of water in greater depth, and there is also a section on water at curezone.com. Bhatmanghelidj recommends, in his book *The Body's Many Cries For Water,* half as many ounces of water per day as pounds of lean weight. Note that for those who claim to drink tons of water but constantly expel large amounts, you are being given a message from your body—and the message is: you have too much garbage inside you! Imagine two five gallon buckets. Both are filled with water, yet one holds the water while the other does not. Why not? It is full of rocks! The body can be glutted with garbage that forces the body to expel its vital water. Clean the kidneys, and use enzymes, enemas, detox methods, oat consumption and oxygen to obtain a healthy water retention.

When fighting infections, note that peroxide is best at the FIRST HINT of an infection, and if taken too late may only be able to hasten recovery by a few days rather than wipe out the illness promptly. Those who avoid refined sugar (perfect fuel for microorganisms and guaranteed to keep them thriving) and load up on natural vitamin C (which improves oxygen levels) while sick will recover fastest. Please try not to drink any soft drinks of any kind when sick--it virtually guarantees a lengthy recovery because of high refined sugar and poor nutrients.

Marc, whose "healing daily" website was linked earlier, states that the common cold can be knocked out within 12-14 hours if a 3% solution of hydrogen peroxide is administered into the ears. He offers evidence gathered suggesting the colds are most likely begun in the ears, and the ears should be the first target gone after.

Oxygen therapy and hydrogen peroxide may seem like ingenious innovations, but one may wonder if the ancient Egyptians would be impressed. An old translation of one of their most comprehensive health remedy lists includes recipes in which honey is featured 50% of the time-and it just so happens that honey is involved in the body's natural synthesis of hydrogen peroxide.

Note that oxygen therapy is only relatively unknown in the US, and has been used extensively with success for decades by thousands all over the globe, especially in Germany, Russia, and Cuba. Ozone therapy has an even more astounding track record in the oxygen annals, but it can also be more expensive. See the aforementioned Pressman material for a superior account, and note that one can get a basic ozone generator for between 250 and 325 dollars at wateroz.com, who also supplies colloidal ionic minerals. Dr. Katz sells a lower power ozone generator at therabreath.com, but it is also less expensive, costing about $110. Ozone generators are almost always worth the money, as one can clean water, clean air, remove odors, and use one of the most powerful of detox procedures—an ozonated water bath, similar to the peroxide bath. One can feel temporarily weak just after an oxygen bath, as the toxins have just been engaged. But once they are controlled, new energy swells.

Bear in mind the central importance of oxygen. Raw foods, with their enzymes, vitamins, minerals, thrive best in clean, oxygen rich water. All cells have an internal engine where oxygen is part of the burning process, unless oxygen levels drop dangerously low, at which point the cells may begin to start fermenting—running the engine in a self defense, besieged mode, with proper cell function deteriorating while the oxygen starvation lasts. Compromising oxygen is like starting a winery in your cellular engines—it only seems sensational until the car crashes.

You can go without food for days. Water must be replenished even sooner. Oxygen? After six minutes with no oxygen in the cells—death results. Think about that.

A note on detoxing for newcomers: a number of people feel better when their toxins are buried in their tissues than when they are being released into the bloodstream. In fact, many folks feel downright lousy when very toxic substances are being freed. And many will actually feel quite good when consuming toxic substances.

So your feelings are a guide, but not the best indicator of your improvement. You really want to know if you are getting better or worse?

Diagnostic methods are tackled next....

5. Diagnostics

As we learn the ways of nutrition, supplements, detox, and oxygen, one may wonder how exactly to evaluate your overall health without any overt sign of stress-are there any tricks we can learn that will give us easy insight into our general health status? Actually, there are countless simple ways to do so cheaply. Dr. Bernard Jensen, mentioned earlier, has written a book called *Visions of Health,* discussing a method whereby overall health can be considered by studying the information encoded into the iris of the eye-a field called iridology. Adam Jackson has written another book in the field called *Iridology,* while Donald Bamer offers yet another called *Practical Iridology And Sclerology.* These methods have their place for the patient with no funds wanting to understand both the troubled parts of their system, and whether or not a given health initiative is working. By looking at various marks and colorations in the eye, the inner status is plainly revealed. The eyes are indeed mirrors. Actually, with the right training, the tongue, the hands, the feet could all be used to evaluate the whole, as everything in the body is very connected. For example, one sign of poor nutrient absorption on the hands is the condition of the nails. Fingernails with vertical striations or toenails with horizontal ones indicate deficiencies—healthy nails should be smoothly rounded.

Another way to assess your health is by paying attention to the colors of your body: healthy blood is bright red, unhealthy blood is darker; healthy urine is clear or light yellow, while poorly hydrated urine is a darker yellow; healthy stools are dark brown and solid, while unhealthier ones are lighter and disintegrate easily, for example.

If your hair is losing color, getting frizzy, and falling out, you are declining; if getting richer, more lustrous, shiny, softer and wavier, you are improving. Note that some may witness freak hair color changes during detox. The body may elect to expel certain toxins through the hair.

Your bowel movements simply must be proportionate to your meals—if they are not, consider correcting this problem to be your number one priority. Though reports conflict on this point, Jennifer Gerhardt (trulyorganicdist@aol.com/ 602-258-1174) states emphatically that stools should float and not sink. She believes that getting your gut bacteria back on track is the way to have healthy stools (and wipe out most diseases, especially mold infections), and an easy way to do this is by making homemade sauerkraut—contact her to find out how. Raw milk also helps.

For a more old fashioned, yet still naturally informative approach, one may wish to try Dr. Loomis' 24 hr. urinalysis to determine nutritional needs. The cost is $65. You mail the sample in and the results are back in a week or so. Call moonlight health at 1- 888-337-0511 to order, available 24 hrs a day. The same group offers Body Balance Mineral Check hair analysis to check levels of 11 important minerals and 9 toxic elements. Saliva analysis is available from the aforementioned alkalize for health website, and from a Dr. Clark trained group: SanaVital@bluewin.ch. The aforementioned alkalize for health site also offers saliva testing. Contact either of them for more info to start forming your own opinions about what is happening inside your body. Dr. Wallach believes hair analysis shows some things other methods cannot, consult his website for more.

So if you really want test results to track which way you are going, there are your options.

An even more powerful insightful tool appears at the end of this book.

6. Therapeutics

Some tools in natural healing are diagnostic, while others are therapeutic. Now let us consider some of the more amazing therapeutic tools available.

Have you ever seen an optometrist gravely instructing another in proper eye care while squinting through spectacles? Did you find that odd? Well, William Bates did, too, and he did something about it. You can find his ideas in a book called *Better Eyesight Without Glasses*. In thousands of cases, schoolchildren in public schools improved to 20/20 vision or better by following his instructions. On the web, you can get an overview of this and other nonlens based approaches to improving vision at I-see.org. Go to the library section for background. In Bates' case, he had found, and in his view shown experimentally, that the essence of poor vision was not muscle strain so much as an overall tension. Once the tension was removed, sight was restored, sometimes, shockingly, within minutes. At the very least, a key forward step in this method is to visit the website, and access a page that has eye charts ready to be printed. Print out a chart, post it on a wall, then read it in the morning first with both eyes, then once with each eye covered, and strive for improvements. One should relax at all times and not strain. Deep breathing can aid this process. There are many further notes to cover here, but they can be found in Bates' brief book, and by starting a voyage from the website just given. You can hopefully have your optometrist change your prescription as you improve.

For those who may find it too difficult to try and leap right away to life without glasses, a step down approach can be employed by learning to use what are often referred to as pinhole reader glasses, which sell for somewhere between 15 and 25 bucks. Often those with even the worst vision can somehow see better when looking through the pinhole glasses, and the eyes are on their way to recovery. This particular research area cries out for more investigators, but those who visit the website and experiment freely will likely find their own best methods with some dedication to this cause.

The aforementioned Stanley Burroughs also mentions eye drops that can help vision in many ways. The drops are made of 5 parts distilled water, 2 parts best grade of honey, 1 part pure apple cider vinegar. They may be applied one at a time to both eyes several times daily. Many cases of glaucoma, cataracts, spots, film and growths have completely disappeared, claims Burroughs. Even if these drops are not tried, it should be mentioned that the better the diet, the better the vision. Many companies like Rockland sell nutrients that can aid the eyes. A great many individuals, after prolonged nutrition with enzymes, vitamins and minerals, witness sharper vision (pun intended), even perfect vision.

And hey, while you are improving your vision so much so cheaply, why not clean your ears while you are at it, with a process called ear coning? Coning, (also called ear candling) is an ancient practice, and involves the painless insertion of a special hollowed candle into the ear. The conee lies on their side, and the candle is placed into the ear, then lit. The flame at the top consumes nearby oxygen, in such a way that a vacuum is created in the hollow candle. The debris clogging the inner ear and sinuses thus is encouraged to exit the body and be trapped in the candle. Be careful not to clear out all the wax. The potential results are not only improved hearing, but sight and overall health improvements depending on the individual (supposedly this can be helpful in some mold infections). Doing the procedure 2 or 3 times the first 2 weeks is recommended. Use your own judgement. For an introduction to this process, please see bibkit.com and click on the ear coning info, or call health stores to see what they have available to you.

The tools just mentioned mainly improve the senses, but other tools mainly help the whole body at once.

The most superior tool of all is, undoubtedly, exercise. Exercise strengthens bones and muscles, as well as the immune system, improves the heart and circulation, increases oxygenation, cleans the lymphatic system, and alters body chemistry, not only by increasing pleasure chemicals like the frequently mentioned endorphins / enkephalins, but also lesser known but equally important neurotransmitters like serotonin.

Moving to more mundane tools, an ancient type of tool that has a mysterious track record of success is the simple magnet. Magnets can be quite cheap or fairly expensive, but they influence circulation and, according to some, can even affect pH levels, with a corresponding effect on health. They also have stunned many of the injured by their unflagging ability to diminish or even banish pain. Two introductory books one can read on the subject are *Healing Magnets* by Sherry Kahn and *Magnet Therapy* by Ghanshyam Birla, but probably the books giving the best overview would be *The Body Magnetic* or *Magnetic Healing* by Buryl Payne, whose website is at buryl.com. The biosouth pole of magnets often stimulates while the bionorth calms. Magnets have not only sped up injury recovery rates, but cheaply improved oxygenation levels, possibly enhanced enzyme activities, and worked wonders in improving joints.

Payne, much like the author of the amazing, yet still neglected new theory of the atom found at polytope.www1.50megs.com, believes strongly in the power of spin as a fundamental natural force. Researcher Manfred Bauer has developed some most extraordinary research which, in the end, enables a positive, constructive, left spin to be imparted to fluids, revitalizing them with potentially astounding results. For background on this seemingly science fictional innovation, read the info at this link: http://www.lifechangetips.com/pri.html . At this time, we would like to see more results from products based on these ideas, but the preliminary results are quite impressive, to say the least. Products may be ordered here more cheaply than the previous link: http://www.holisticfamilyandpets.com/mall/water2.htm.

One of the mightiest health pioneers in recent years is Dr. Hulda Clark, who has written the aforementioned book *The Cure For All Diseases,* as well as *The Cure For All Cancers* and

The Cure For Hiv/Aids. Her information is so voluminous we have time only to mention a few pieces of it here. One of her most critical breakthroughs is an electronic device called the zapper, which her books show you how to build yourself for about 25 dollars (one can also order one from her for the cost of a hundred and fifty dollars or so). The zapper delivers a small amount of electricity that often cannot even be felt at all and which executes many pesky little buggers infecting us. It was recently proven clinically to wipe out cancer cells, though it works as well for a legion of nasty critters. It is a fantastic achievement. Dr. Robert Beck has a similar device (indeed, some view the zapper as being derivative of the Beck device, but there appear to be no circuit diagrams of the latter). Dr. Clark also offers a diagnostic tool called a syncrometer which one can use to track results, if you wish.

Some are skeptical of zappers, but there is a litmus test: if you get tired from a zap, you killed pathogens, and the more tired you are, the more pathogens you killed. Healthy people often feel no tiredness at all. Dr. Clark cautions that zappers cannot reach into the bowel or into the recesses of the mouth, where many pathogens lurk. She offers her own strategies to keep these areas clean in her books, but zapping all by itself should not be understood as the solution to all problems. Zappers work best in conjunction with a superior nutritional regimen, such as described in this book. While Clark talks about zapping even for the common cold, those with proper nutrition may expect to simply never have a common cold again! Sickness is not natural, not helpful exercise for the immune system, but a sign of gross errors made.

It may seem a rather ingenious innovation to use electricity to solve health problems, but one may wonder whether the ancient Greeks would be as shocked as we are, pardon the pun. After all, they did capture electric eels from the sea and kept them handy for their own version of the zapper!

Dr. Clark is well aware of oxygen therapies (which is why she sells the right kind of peroxide at her site), and much of the material already presented here. She has also joined the ranks of the many who have found colloidal silver to be effective in battling pathogens. Many microbes, as reinforced by Dr Robert Becker in his book *Cross Currents,* malfunction and die when presented with silver in a certain water soluble colloidal form. Not only that, but a whole legion of maladies can be wiped out by this potent weapon. There are many ways of obtaining colloidal silver. One man claims to be able to do it dirt cheap by attaching wires to ordinary silvered coins dunked in water—as described in this concise background story at http://cat007.com/silver.htm (your eyes may bulge at the constructive possibilities from just one of the methods in this book—intriguing to imagine them in combination). Search the web and choose from countless options, including Dr Clark's site, and the oft mentioned reachforlife.com website of Rockland, phone number 1-800-258-5028. Be warned that some argue that colloidal silver can deactivate both good and bad bacteria. Whenever you target bacteria indiscriminately for elimination, at least be wise enough to be ready to resupply the good bacteria after using a destructive approach.

The Clark methods are some of the most powerful man has yet seen, granting us the ability to beat cancer, aids, diabetes, multiple sclerosis, innumerable health conditions, and do so much more. Her devices could be used to purify the food and water supply, and any manufacturing process we please, for example-the choices are boundless.

Another simple therapeutic tool is plain old vinegar. Many with skin fungal infections found them gone with brief daily dabs or soaks of vinegar. Its health and home uses can be quite extensive, as these links show: http://mdmd.essortment.com/healthbenefit_rmxi.htm and http://frugalliving.about.com/cs/tips/a/vinegar.htm

When we are motivated enough to use them, we now have the tools at our disposal to create a planet of healthy, beautiful, clean individuals—clean in mind and body. Dr. Wallach goes so far as to say there are no geniuses or amazing genetic athletes—only those with sound nutrition histories. We already know alcoholics have poor sperm from their habit, and the evidence mounts that sperm and egg quality are affected by more than just alcohol. The cleaner we are, the more likely it is our children will be toxin-free, healthy, smart and beautiful.

The main tools to create this paradise have now been given to you.

What will *you* do with them?

7. Corruption

It may be difficult for some of you to believe that such powerful methods exist, that some of them have been around for decades, and yet you have never heard of them. If they work so well, why are they not being lauded universally by the media? Is it actually possible that some forces exist which would prefer to profit from death and disease rather than eliminate them?

Consider an incident that happened to Max Gerson, the nutritional pioneer. Once, several decades ago, when the US Congress met to have yet another one of its useless wars, as it often does to wage futile skirmishes against poverty, drugs, or crime, it actually had a decent plan-let Max Gerson testify about his successful outcomes. Witnesses were brought to show his victories, heaps of documentation were offered to prove his case. Congress listened quietly, and a press conference was to follow. We can imagine Dr. Gerson's anticipation that he might be able to share his successes with the world.

But then something happened after his testimony. Representatives from the drug companies sent stooges to the press conference, and invited the reporters away to a party, and told them it would be silly to bother listening to this strange man who actually thought food had an effect on health. Under the relentless pressure, all but one reporter left.

The man who stayed listened, and listened carefully. The ideas made sense to him, and he soon got on the radio to broadcast his findings. The station switchboard lit up with callers eager to know more-until the drug companies found out what was going on. Promptly they called the radio station manager. They reminded him exactly how many millions of dollars in advertising they provided, and that that money could be pulled in an instant should these broadcasts be allowed to continue.

The result was that no further word about Gerson's work was heard again, and the reporter was fired from his job two weeks later.

If you think this is an isolated incident, you are mistaken. Harry Hoxsey was an herbal pioneer. His father once saw his horse getting sick, and soon realized the horse had cancer. But then, strangely, the horse began to get better. Curious as to what miracle was happening with his horse, Hoxsey decided to follow it around and watch what it was doing. He found that it consistently ate from an unusual patch of plants. Intrigued, Hoxsey studied those plants, and began conducting experiments with the herbs therein.

That was when he began to see people being cured of cancer. Among the herbs he used were red clover, buckthorn bark, burdock root, stilingia root, berberis root, pokeberries and root, licorice root, cascara amarga, and prickly ash bark. Potassium iodide was also included, and it is interesting to note that potassium is a key part of the Gerson therapy, as is iodine for its role in assisting the thyroid which is often weakened in ill patients. Of further interest is that some of the aforementioned ingredients are featured prominently in some current bowel cleanse products. An internal tonic and external dressing were developed. John Hoxsey passed this knowledge onto his son Harry.

The medical system would not just believe the herbal stories they were later told-they wanted proof. So Harry Hoxsey gave it to them. He brought one of their supposedly terminal cases back to life. But instead of welcoming this breakthrough, Morris Fishbein, head of the AMA, squashed the whole method with his power and influence, with the result that the method was driven out of the US by 1963.

The story of Dr. Wallach was already given above. Price's research appears to have been buried along with Pottenger's, and is rarely mentioned in the mainstream media today. Pioneers in oxygen therapy have had their facilities besieged with SWAT teams. One oxygen innovator was hacked to death by machetes.

A lecturer on Rife, described below, was killed before delivering a lecture to college students. Another innovator, Wilhelm Reich, saw many of his energy collecting devices smashed to pieces, and was himself thrown in prison. Naessens, described above, was put on trial for helping his fellow man, as was Dinshah Ghadiali, described below.

A hard copy of this book sent to a publisher disappeared, as apparently did the email advising the distributor of its arrival, as apparently were several other emails related to this publication, all without error messages of any kind, while some people associated with this work have been openly threatened.

The situation has actually become so perverse today that some of the most brilliant health pioneers have been targeted as fraudulent by the government in what is tastelessly called *Operation Cure All.*

Today, with every issue, *Nexus* magazine dares to reveal more of these suppressed heroic stories, year after year, while "rebel" news networks like rense.com, conspiracyplanet.com, and davidicke.com challenge the mainstream news networks regarding the truth found by scientific experimentation.

Today, the drug industry represents a 36 billion dollar force (at least), where as much as $300,000 can be drained from each cancer victim. Could it be its goal is to keep itself alive, not its consumers? Jon Rappaport certainly exposes much corruption in his book entitled, *AIDS, inc.*

Many have spoken out assertively against the abuses of modern medicine, such as Robert Mendelsohn in his book *Confessions of a Medical Heretic*-and just like Mendelsohn, they quickly found themselves in a coffin.

Some adults who look at life with a childlike naivete may find it hard to believe that not all villains wear black, have overt fangs and speak of evil, and that some of them actually wear suits and ties, smile warmly and speak of peace. Then again, some children learn this lesson by the time they are six years old.

It does not matter if some think this debate of those who favor pure nature versus warped nature cannot be settled by the common man, because the common man lacks sufficient education and sophisticated tools to reach an independent conclusion. The time for letting so called experts decide everything for us is past. It is past because you are reading this book. The tools in this book are so cheap it is now all too easy for you to verify whether the information presented here is false or correct. Nearly every idea in this book can be tested individually for the cost of one visit to the office of a drugloving doctor, and those that cannot can certainly be tested far more easily than the cost of a drug lord treatment for any serious illness.

In the end, it is not the clothes worn, the cost of an education, the prestige of a journal where articles were published, or how many syllables in the vocabulary words that can be stretched out of a mouth that counts.

From now on, truth can be defined in one way, and one way alone, the way science always should have defined it: by the results obtained by simple experiments anyone can duplicate.

From now on, it is up to *you*.

8. Rife

Thus far we have seen that health is largely a matter of nutrition and purity in the environment and self. Many people striving to recover from health problems can grow frustrated, however, from a seeming lack of mathematical precision in health methods. For example, with some of the tools of natural healing, there may seem to be a little variation in the results. One may take an herb, and find that it works better for a friend than it does for you. One may take an enzyme, and find that it works better for you than for your friend. Melatonin and oxygen can sometimes take days to work fully. Clark's zappers do work quickly, but because they work via electricity, there sometimes can be a snag as electricity appears to travel around the outside of the organs and may not penetrate mostly hollow places such as the intestine, where many parasites lurk. As mentioned before, cleaning the colon can solve the last problem, but even so, some pathogens hide in areas under our teeth, and these can be hard to reach. Is there any way to penetrate the body completely and give the pathogens *no* safe hiding place?

Indeed there is.

One of the greatest unsung geniuses of history was a man named Royal Raymond Rife, whose story is described not only in *Suppressed Inventions* but in the book *The Cancer Cure That Worked,* by Barry Lynes. Rife not only succeeded in proving that cancer was caused by pathogens, but he also showed that he could destroy those pathogens, 100% of the time. How did he do it? With a principle known as destructive resonance.

Resonance comes from root words which translate as "to sound again". A common example of resonance is when an opera star shatters a glass with her voice. The glass has its own sound frequency, and when the opera star matches that sound with her voice, or sounds the note again, there is resonance. Waves build up in the glass until such time as the particles of the glass are driven apart with those waves, and destruction results. The brilliant electrical pioneer Nikola Tesla once proved that he could even destroy buildings with a device based on destructive resonance.

Resonance in a more constructive form is also the essence of the Clark analytical tool called the syncrometer. Each microbe emits a frequency. It is possible to build a simple electrical circuit openly described in the Clark literature, with two test probes. One probe may be placed over a lab prepared sample of a given pathogen, and the other probe directed close to the body where a pathological presence may be suspected. If there is resonance, detected as a little tickle or tingle in the fingers holding the test probe, the presence of a given pathogen is confirmed.

Royal Raymond Rife used this same principle of resonance, in its destructive form, to show he could kill pathogens.

First he developed a microscope that defied the laws of physics as understood at the time. Today, most optical or lightbased microscopes can at best manage 2,000 times magnification. Rife managed 60,000 times. He saw things that perhaps no one else had seen before in history. Once he had identified cancer pathogens, he proved that he could use destructive resonance to shatter them, 100% of the time. He repeated his tests 400 times in a row with the same unmistakably successful result.

There was a celebration at the time, back in the 1930's, and a newspaper headline shouted that it was the end of all disease.

But then the drug companies zoomed in. You can guess the rest.

One might say that this story is too incredible. Is there any way we can see the same results today somehow? Does anyone actually have film footage of microbes being destroyed by frequencies?

The answer is yes. James Bare, a man who studied the work of Rife, has built a device very similar to the original Rife device. Undoubtedly he could have built an identical one had the precise plans ever been made publicly available. Bare's device works with plasma rather than electricity. Still, the results are the same. From his website at rt66.com/-rifetech/ (the wavy line is the little squiggle in the upper left of your keyboard), you may order a videotape which will show you, in no uncertain terms, film footage of various microorganisms as they are first slowed down, then destroyed when their cell walls are ruptured and their innards spill out into the surrounding environment. This happens repeatedly, so all that a skeptic has to do is get some popcorn and watch. For those who simply wish to experiment with devices of this type, some are sold at Jaguar enterprises, and many other devices out there are based on the same principles, such as those sold by Cherry Maly. You may search the net by typing in keywords like 'rife frequency machines' and make your choices. These types of frequency machines tend to be far more costly than zappers, more complicated, and sometimes less efficient. One should try to learn the details of what each process involves before making a commitment.

Hulda Clark has also joined the frequency bandwagon, and has recently offered a relatively cheap frequency generator called the minifg. See her website at drclark.net for more.

Frequency work can be done in many ways. One way is for the frequencies to be carried in a waveform called a square wave. A square wave is so named because when its signal is sent into a device called an oscilloscope, the display shows a waveform that looks like a square. But other waveforms can be used, and in different ways.

For example, another way of working with frequencies is to help establish healthy frequencies for various organs. Not only do microorganisms have frequencies, but so do our kidneys, lungs, liver and all the rest. It is possible to construct a frequency waveform in such a way that the targeted organ is positively and constructively stimulated to heal, rather than destruct. Not long ago, Julie Clemens, a naturopathic doctor, actually got approval from the FDA for a device to deliver these helpful frequencies.

She offers frequencies to restore inner organs, regrow hair, repair skin, gums and countless other conditions. One of her cheapest models is $1,000 and can be used on a home computer. The amperage of the current is so low that, much like the zapper, one cannot feel anything when the device is on. The potential in this field is almost unlimited.

9. Spectrochrome

For those who find the electrical approach not to their liking for whatever reason, there is yet another way to go with frequency that is cheaper, if not faster: spectrochrome therapy.

Dinshah Ghadiali (use the keyword dinshah) eventually found his way from India to the US, where he pioneered in the use of colored light to heal clients. To this day Dinshah remains a favorite target of the drug lords, who seem to cherish mocking the man who claims light frequencies can heal. A typical joke is to say, "How can this possibly work? It is just lights!"

Nevertheless, one of the greatest marvels in all of nature is the process of photosynthesis where plants make food after converting energy from-what? Just light, of course. And how does the human body manufacture vitamin D, which is important in the body's absorption of calcium? Why, with just light. How is it that the pineal gland in the brain knows when to deliver its doses of the all important melatonin? By paying attention to "just light". To act as if light is meaningless and useless is not only unscientific, but in itself piteously daft.

Dinshah worked with his lights for years, and taught his methods to any who were interested. One woman who was interested was Kate Baldwin, a medical doctor in Philadelphia. She incorporated spectrochrome in her therapy, and became so happy with it she claimed that she preferred using spectrochrome first over any other method. One such case was particularly amazing. A young girl was brought to her hospital with very severe third degree burns. Her skin was blackened from fire, and her condition critical. Asking her superior what she could do in this case, Dr. Baldwin was saddened to hear him say that in a case this drastic, there was nothing to be done--death was the only conclusion to wait for. Refusing to accept this, Dr. Baldwin turned once again to spectrochrome. The girl did not die. 18 months later, her skin was almost fully restored, and in the Dinshah book, *Let There Be Light* there are pictures one can see from this case. In addition, there is a transcript of the courtroom testimony of Dr. Baldwin supporting spectrochrome-the case is on record-- which anyone can verify whenever they please.

Dinshah developed protocols to improve countless health conditions, diabetes, endometriosis, multiple sclerosis, (cancer of course) high blood pressure, and an endless stream of others. But even if one did not see a particular disease or condition listed in his book, this should not prevent them from using spectrochrome. There are patterns in the use of the colors that one can use to make intelligent guesses as to which colors to try for a given condition. It is hard to fault this method for its price: a basic set of filters, giving you basically all you need, would be a mere $35 or so. One can use almost any light source for the initial light, even sunlight, which at the time of this book's creation is still free. To order a filter pack, call this number in Texas: 214-421-0757. You may also visit the Dinshah website at dinshahhealth.org.

It became evident from this work, and other work similar to it, such as that done in Kirlian photography, that there does indeed exist what is called the human energy field, or aura. Spectrochrome works by influencing this aura, which then influences the body. To state that there is an aura does not necessarily mean that the energy in this aura is some new or exotic form of energy, but perhaps one of so fine a frequency our instruments are not fully capable of grasping it as yet.

Dr Robert Becker, in his books titled *The Body Electric* and *Cross Currents,* revealed that acupuncture and acupressure do not influence a vague system of energy in the human body, but rather a very specific one that he himself helped to define in more precise terms.

Classically, when neurologists, who study the brain, spoke of brain cell activity, they tended to focus on neurons, or nerve cells, generally dismissing the fact that in the brain, neurons are the least popular kind. Rather, glial cells and other seemingly useless structural cells dominate, though little attention was paid to their function. Becker helped us to understand that while the neurons did indeed represent a very clever digital form of processing information, the support cells represented an equally impressive, but fundamentally simpler method of processing information via a direct current analog system. It is this DC analog system that can be shown via real scientific instruments to have power lines running through the body, which the Chinese and all those who have been using acupuncture/acupressure have been harmonizing for centuries while the rest of the world waits to wake up. There was once a report of a man encased in ice who had the meridian lines tattooed across his body. We seem forever haunted by the possibilities of what the ancients knew.

Dr. John Whitman Ray, in Australia, has developed a method of combining iridology, acupressure, correct diet via juicing of rockdust grown plants, oxygen therapies, and more to accomplish what he terms body regeneration. To totally understand his work requires the purchasing of videotapes that cost hundreds of dollars, but at least you have still another possibility to explore. His website is: bodyelectronics.com. Do not expect to contact Dr. Ray directly however, as he was killed under mysterious circumstances before opening a cancer clinic in Australia.

Wilhelm Reich, whose story is also mentioned in suppressed inventions, also worked with this energy of the body. One of the most fascinating, but perhaps poorly understood, aspects of Reich's work concerned the orgasm and its relationship to health. Reich became convinced that the orgasm was vital to rejuvenating the life energy, and observed a consistent pattern in his cancer patients of an unfulfilling sex life seeming to be a precondition to their diseased states. In some ways, it appears the orgasm acts as a release of the old stagnant energy, allowing in the fresh new energy. Could life be suggesting that those who live best also enjoy it the most? Or is that too radical an idea?

Just to be clear, before any get too overenthusiastic about this function of the orgasm, it should be pointed out that excessive orgasms can drain the life energy. (It is curious that Buryl Payne's notes on magnetism seem to reinforce this notion, as rodents in cages surrounded by a magnetic field lived longer, as if they were storing charge, but only lived longer if not allowed to copulate.)

Already in this book you have learned how to practically wipe out every major disease known to man, how to stimulate the body's inner organs to health, and even how a burn victim given up for dead was restored to full life. How much more can we do?

Well, how unlimited is *your* imagination?

10. Bioacoustics

Napolean Hill once wrote "whatever the mind of man can conceive and believe, it can achieve." So next let us consider what may well be the most inspiring of all healing methods and perhaps the most tantalizing of all forms of energy frequencies: the bioacoustics of Sharry Edwards.

As we have already established, frequencies in the form of electricity, plasma and light can bring about dramatic changes in the human condition. In the same way, there is yet another form in which these frequencies may attain their effects: sound.

The light frequencies of spectrochrome correspond to sound frequencies as notes in a diatonic musical scale. The color red, for example, can be shown as equivalent to the musical note of C. If you deliver a sound wave on the appropriate frequency, the brain shall process this information and make changes accordingly. It is even possible to influence the body to produce the minerals it needs, simply by supplying the body with the frequency of that mineral. For example, calcium has a frequency which is the musical equivalent of the note E. Thus, an octave of E can be delivered to the brain and calcium can manifest in the body. In just this way, osteoporosis can be reversed. Sound, insofar as its waves can be programmed to hundredths of a hertz, can be more precise than light in effecting change.

Sharry Edwards made these and a great many other similar observations, and she has packaged them in a rigidly scientific and technological way, called Bioacoustics. By use of either a sophisticated piano tuner or proprietary software, Sharry and her trained practitioners can analyze a 45 second voice print and gain a vocal spectral analysis to determine which notes are in stress, and exactly what frequencies are out of balance in a given individual. Based on this information, she can prescribe sound frequencies in a very specific waveform for input to a given individual until such time as the brain is trained and the assistance is no longer necessary. The ideal is a voice balanced on all frequencies.

Extending herself, in recent years, Sharry has proven that she can dissolve the protein coat of pathogens with sound, effectively ripping off their disguises and exposing them as the invaders that they are to our immune system, who promptly shows them the door. She can also weaken and strengthen a given muscle, again with sound frequencies. In the case of her son, who had suffered a terrible motorcycle accident and had his patella or kneecap removed, she was actually able to regenerate the patella, 3/4 of the way at last notice. In another case, Sharry was able to predict thyroid trouble for a gentleman. He went to a hospital for a second opinion, but the hospital could find no problem with any of its tools, and wondered if there were any merit to this cutting edge approach. Less than a week later, the man collapsed. The origin of his problem was a thyroid condition. The voice analysis saw things conventional medicine could not.

This work is so amazing that it has actually had an impact on those with Down's syndrome. After being presented with sound, a boy suffering from Down's was able to show improved math skills within hours. Bioacoustics can even go so far as to show if a physical problem has its origin in the emotions, or vice versa. Just how far can this technology go? Perhaps your action or lack thereof after listening to this tape will be the deciding factor.

In some ways bioacoustics can help us solve problems we cannot even yet name. In the process of correcting imbalanced frequencies, we may correct problems we cannot yet define.

More provocative still, Edwards' research has indicated that each person has their own musical scale, if you will. What harmonizes with a given individual can be determined by using a formula that relates their notes to the notes of various substances.

Thus we may at last have a precise insight as to why the effects of foods and medications vary so much from person to person.

Not only that, but bioacoustics may be used to evaluate the effectiveness of every other method mentioned in this book.

There are further ramifications to this astounding new work in frequency. In the same way that music theory shows that certain frequencies of notes sound harmonious when expressed together, the evidence begins to suggest that we each have principal note frequencies, and that our compatibility with others may be significantly influenced by frequencies surrounding us of which we may not be consciously aware, but rather speak of in common slang as good or bad vibes. Could it be that all this time we have been speaking of a literal truth?

For more information on the Bioacoustics of Sharry Edwards, please contact sound health at soundhealthinc.com, or call 740-698-9119.

By the way, using sound for health might seem like a rather ingenious innovation, but those monks chanting in long drawn out notes in ancient Tibet might not be so impressed...

11. Attitude

While we are on the subject of attitude, quite possibly no survey of natural healing would be complete without reference to the importance of keeping a positive mental attitude while healing. There is little doubt that emotions have a profound effect on healing, in quite scientific ways. For example, consider the case of bed wetting in children. The evidence strongly suggests that bed wetters are low in potassium. But potassium levels are often regulated by the adrenal glands resting atop the kidneys. The adrenal glands release substances that are the biochemical expressions of our emotions; for example, adrenaline may be considered fear, and noradrenaline anger. Thus, for some children frequently exposed to situations which fill them with fear, their adrenal glands can become exhausted, and their potassium levels then drop, and bedwetting may be the result.

In the case of candida, scientists claim that stress means cortisol production, and the candida can feed off the cortisol—which means if you are going into stress, maintain as positive an attitude as possible, or the bad microorganisms will feed off your cortisol!

Yet while many frequently point to the role of emotions in health, much less attention is paid to the idea that our emotions stem from our beliefs. Two may witness the same incident, and one might laugh where the other cries. The event itself does not automatically project its own emotion, but rather, the emotion arises from our interpretation of what we experience. It follows that those with the depth to respond with love rather than hate, and courage rather than fear, shall be constructively orchestrating the biochemical environment of the body with respect to health.

In recent times it has become almost fashionable to talk about the belief some have that we each create our own reality from our minds. While a simple experiment may show quite vividly that wishing does not make it so, consider the following experiment as an alternative.

A young boy, as a child, used to watch a woman often play classic solitaire. To be sure, she seemed quite proud of her intelligence, yet seemed to win only about 10% of the time, if that. He suspected that if asked, she would have stated most assuredly that she played well, and sometimes you just lose.

The boy grew to read the writings of Galileo, in which Galileo stated, "It is not always profitable to do everything that lies within one's power." As a man, the player had occasion to revisit classic solitaire, and studied it more closely. He found that a majority of losses came from leaving the last two large piles untapped. He then began ignoring certain plays he could make in an effort to ensure he could minimize those last two piles. His winning percentage increased to about 50%.

Studying the game more closely, he found ways of anticipating several plays ahead, knowing where all cards would be after he made several moves, making moves that left several options open, and subtle tricks that the casual eye would miss. His percentage increased to about 80% wins.

But after all he had learned, there still seemed to be some deals of the cards that were unwinnable—situations where no plays could be made—a complete dead end—or was it?

We are all confronted each day of our lives with what we are told is a meaningless, random series of events—but is this really the case? A guitar may make any kind of noise when played, but will only make music when attuned...

The player tried an experiment on the computer. Before hitting the "deal" command, he paused, filled himself up with the most constructive vision of harmony he could think of, wished for a winning outcome, then hit the button.

His winning percentage increased to 100%.

Might all of life be this way? Many might eagerly focus on the positive benefits of the mental attitude in this story, completely glossing over the knowledge that provided the foundation to the winning track record—but could success not be the ultimate blending of hard work to understand the pattern, coupled with an intention of manifesting beauty and harmony?

Try for yourself and see...

Still another aspect of attitude that cries out for notice from human experience is the often lethal risk involved in constantly and lazily assuming that responsibility for our health and understanding its maintenance does not belong to us but rather to some outside expert. Perhaps life is absurdly complicated and we must forever pay millions for verbose and ultimately alien explanations of everyday events. Or perhaps, nature radiates a constant and steady grace, willing to share its beauty with absolutely anyone with the guts and receptivity to just look. Perhaps responsibility for your health has been, is and always will be, your sole responsibility, and your own skills are very much the result of nothing more than the sum total of times you dare to learn just a little bit more.

For more books on belief systems and health, you may wish to read the writings of Norman Cousins, such as the classic *Anatomy of an Illness,* or perhaps *Head First: The Biology of Hope.* For more on constructive belief systems, you may wish to peruse Richard Bach and his books like *Jonathan Livingston Seagull* and *Illusions,* Maxwell Maltz and his book *Psycho-cybernetics,* the writings of Wayne Dyer, and even *Walden And Other Writings* by Henry Thoreau.

And to understand and empower yourself to appreciate the beauty, elegance and wonders of nature all about you, you may wish to take a basic science tour of your world with books like *Makers of Mathematics* by Alfred Hooper, *Conceptual Physical Science* by Paul Hewitt, *Anatomy and Physiology* by Rod Seeley, *Patterns in Nature* by Peter Stevens, *The Self Made Tapestry* by Philip Ball, and *A Beginner's Guide to Constructing the Universe* by Michael Schneider.

When you do not know the way your world works, you can feel isolated, afraid and impotent. But when you are empowered those feelings can change until you feel connected, radiant, and powerful—a spirit in harmony with all that exists.

Which do you prefer?

12. Regeneration

Debate on ultimate health methods has gone on for centuries, possibly millennia, but if you want to settle the debate once and for all that the methods presented here are the best, you will not need to consult a fifty mile long bibliography, purchase multimillion dollar particle accelerators or pray for divine visitation—but you will have to perform a simple task that no other health methods have ever been able to do: erase any "permanent" skin damage.

Of the pioneers presented in this book, four have accomplished regeneration to some extent: Becker, by using specialized electrical equipment most people will likely never have access to; Ghadiali, whose spectrochrome is easily accessible but has apparently limited effects; Dr. Ray, who has seen some body regeneration but whose practitioners want $65 for the privilege of talking to them and stress their methods must be used by specialists only; Sharry Edwards' bioacoustics, which also requires great expense, time and reliance on others.

But what if you had the power to completely eradicate a permanent scar? Utterly erase any stretch mark, no matter how many years old? Cure baldness, no matter how long it had been in effect? And what if you could do all these things by yourself, dirt cheap? Would it not then seem you had attained a higher level of mastery in natural healing than the greatest experts in history?

Well, now you can.

The research in this manual has transformed over time, and led any who followed it to its own inevitable direction. That direction shows that to accomplish ultimate healing, we need ultimate nutrition.

Therefore, if cells are not healing, they are not getting total nutrition. We can prove what total nutrition is by simply taking some "permanently" damaged skin—and repairing it completely.

Totally repairing skin is one of the toughest healing challenges there is, one that leaves nearly all investigators giving up in resignation. Digesting the right nutrients seems unlikely to solve the matter, simply because when skin is severely damaged, its blood vessel supply is also damaged. No supply line—no repair.

In addition, the nerve supply is usually also shot, taking the brain effectively out of the crisis loop. If the brain is unaware of a problem, it does nothing to fix it.

Some researchers, understanding this, opted for an alternate strategy—apply nutrients directly to a damaged skin area. But this approach nearly always failed as well. Why? The skin, among other things, is a defensive barrier—a protector of our insides. It does not allow many substances to pass through its hallowed gates. Countless molecules enter, precious few can penetrate. So if you cannot get in through the blood, and skin is generally too hard to break through, how do you get in?

Answer: by developing a total nutritional formula with a small particle size that the body will immediately recognize as useful, and allow to wholly penetrate. And thus is the Totaloe formula announced for the first time in this book.

The base of the formula is aloe vera—"the great healer". Researchers have already noted for some time that aloe vera has the power to penetrate all skin layers. For this reason alone it might be chosen to carry other nutrients. But its penetration power is more than chance. In and of itself, aloe vera is rich in nutrients: containing an abundance of electrolytic major minerals, vitamins like a, b's, and c, amino acids and even fatty acids. Thus it is primed to recharge the meridians all by itself, and is eagerly welcomed by the body. It would appear this electrical charging capacity may be critical to the restoration of innervation and blood vessel supply to damaged areas. Small wonder that aloe vera is one of the first and best choices for application to burned skin.

If you apply aloe vera to many damaged skin tissues, you may see them heal partially or even completely. But there are variations in results—why?

The quality of the aloe vera would explain it. In order to test a more complete aloe vera, the Totaloe formula was designed, by adding Rockland's Liquid Life to an aloe vera base. The present Totaloe formula described here is equal parts raw aloe vera juice and Liquid Life. When this formula hits the skin, amazing things happen.

Though these experiments are brand new, here are some preliminary results:

A man with a permanent scar on his knuckle watched it slowly disappear over months.

A soccer player with shins contaminated from shin guards saw skin damaged for 15 years completely heal.

A body builder with stretch marks on his sides from leg pressing 800 pounds saw the marks completely disappear.

A balding man saw hair follicles dead for 15 years immediately come back to life. Not all hairs came back at once, but the declining areas resurged first, then the dead areas began to stir, until even completely dead areas were renewed.

A bodybuilder with blood vessel damage in his arm saw the vessels visibly return to normal after being damaged nearly ten years.

So if you have any of these problems, or any skin problem that does not appear to be improving otherwise, test Totaloe—it seems the cells of the body have no choice but to respond to complete nutrition. No multimillion dollar machinery needed, no tokamaks or 24x36 spread sheets charting subatomic particle interactions—just aloe vera with a few cheap, extra nutrients.

How about that.

A note from these experiments is in order—*the fresher the aloe vera, the more potent*. The gel in the center of the leaves is considered the main healing liquid, but experiments show that the whole can be even more effective if you juice the whole leaves (after cutting off the jagged sides) and include the chlorophyll in your formula. Chlorophyll's healing properties are already well known, and since magnesium is at its core, it is just that much more of an electrolytic boost to the whole. Aloe vera grows quickly and easily—all the more reason to prepare it yourself, especially since you can water it with peroxide and mineralize its soil for maximum effect. *The best way to work with Totaloe is to make only as you much as you will use at once.* It will still work if stored—but more slowly.

Experiments are underway to see if Totaloe can regenerate teeth, and to see if it can regrow the amputated leg of a dog—there is no reason for it to fail in either case.

The results will appear in future editions.

What are the limits of Totaloe? Are there any? Can the blind be made to see? The deaf to hear? Could severe burn victims return to normal? Perhaps your experiments will tell us.

The simplest Totaloe formula has not yet been decided upon. The aloe vera in these experiments, while raw, was not grown with rock dust. Would aloe with rock dust accomplish all these results by itself? Future experiments will tell.

Earlier in the book, certain kinds of regeneration were mentioned, such as restoring hair color. Dr. Wallach points out that hair color loss is primarily a mineral deficiency—then is the most effective way to solve this problem by supplementing heavily with the apparently low minerals (copper, sulfur)?

The research presented here, in moving on, begins to lean more heavily in a new direction. Even better than supplementing with large quantities of a deficient nutrient appears to be the strategy of cleansing the body first, then letting the body use small quantities of the deficient nutrient with great efficiency.

In the detox chapter you were given a great many detox strategies, and if used properly, all can be outstanding in detoxing the body. But it is interesting to note that one method mentioned in passing in the oxygen chapter may be indeed be the most powerful detox method: working with the liquid oxygen product from Rockland. Experiments have shown it not only equal in power to 35% food grade peroxide, but better. Given the ingredients, this is not surprising. For example, the product contains a selenium amino acid chelate. This chelate enhances the activity of the body's naturally occurring oxygenation enzymes.

Detox can be quite a graphic process. One of the most telltale signs of detox is a change in the appearance of the tongue. Provided you do have toxins in you, your tongue will, in all likelihood, change in texture and color as you detox. So one graphic way to ascertain whether you have purged virtually all toxins would be: start on a liquid oxygen product, watch the tongue worsen in appearance as the toxins are engaged, and when the tongue returns to normal, detox is done.

Another sign to watch for in detox is heavy bags under the eyes. This usually means the kidneys are getting hit hard with the burden of trying to neutralize the toxins oxygen has expelled from certain bodily hiding places. Some detox products on the market are so powerful you do run a risk of expelling more toxins than the body can cope with effectively—obviously you do not want to intensify detox beyond your point to cope. So detox at what feels like a comfortable rate for you. Remember fresh watermelon will help your kidneys if they are getting roughed up during detox. Also remember to support your liver as described in the detox chapter. Some who find themselves coughing when detox is started may especially profit from supporting the liver—it seems herbs like silymarin and cayenne can grab the toxins in such a way that the body chooses not to force coughing on the subject.

Interestingly, Rockland's oxygen product is rich in aloe vera. Potentially this oxygenation process can clean and even regenerate every internal organ.

Some may wonder if cleaning the insides will help clean the outsides. Certainly cleaning oneself inside cannot help but improve the outside. This is because cleaning the inside will clean the blood, therefore any skin area receiving a better blood supply can potentially improve. But can blood vessel repair and nerve regeneration take place in damaged superficial skin from orally ingested nutrients alone? At present the answer is unknown.

The new theory of regeneration emerging here is that for regeneration to take place, blood vessels and nerves must be regenerated, and this can be done in special ways. While most argue that this is impossible, you have been presented with five different ways of doing it in this book. Each method works with energy in one form or another, and it is this energy which seems to prod blood vessels and nerves to regenerate. The Totaloe formula seems to trigger regeneration in the manner most harmonious with nature: electrical energy (what Becker showed to be dc analog) is developed in weakened areas by saturating those areas with electrolytes—electrical carrier minerals like calcium.

The working hypothesis for now will be: *any damaged area can eventually heal, if provided with energy in the right form.*

Undoubtedly there are many who are wholly indifferent to the possibilities of regrowing limbs and demand to know if the nutritional formulas can do more important things, like get rid of wrinkles. Future experiments will prove if this can be done, but there is no reason to believe that wrinkles would not succumb to nutrition as well. What is important to bear in mind is that *the greater the damage, the longer the repair time.*

While all problems will likely improve immediately, complete repair may take months, and, in some cases, possibly years. The more nature is harmonized with, the faster the success.

But it should be expected that every problem state, for those not seconds away from certain death, can not only be improved, but given enough time, utterly eliminated.

Now for those who, in the pursuit of perfection, wonder about the possibilities not merely of returning a youthful status quo, but perhaps improving upon it, there are a few notes.

Some women, for example, spend fortunes on breast enhancement, and wonder if nature can offer any help in this regard. Of course it can!

First, all must understand that hormones, the primary regulators of growth, are not in the genetic code (though the enzymes that influence them are). Given that no hormone can be constructed without the individual consuming the appropriate fatty acids, there is no such thing as a human whose genes alone led to flawless sexual development regardless of essential fatty acids consumed!

One way sexual development might be safely attained, as described previously, is by consuming the dairy products of live fed (not dry fed) animals, richly oxygenated as described McCabe, whose food comes from a mineral and generally nutrient rich soil.

But for those women who wonder about other options, there are certain herbal combinations one may experiment with. For female hormones, many have found combinations of fenugreek, saw palmetto, wild yam, and fennel to work well. Some companies interestingly tack on herbs that have nothing to do with hormone regulation, but are known to help the liver or the bowel. If you have read the previous chapters, this makes sense. So many will say, not just in breast enhancement cases, but in trying countless health methods, individual results vary, and shruggingly leave it at that. But let us at least point out that of all factors that vary, the most important one that prevents success is likely this: *how much garbage does the failing individual have inside them?* A prerequisite for success in such cases is likely nothing more than a thorough detoxing of garbage. Once that is done, if one then consumes the *complete* nutrition described in this book, success should be assured. In any case, those who try herbal preparations along these lines to either ease period pain, stabilize hormones, or enhance breasts, please email what works for you to the email at the end of this book, so others can know your results.

We should never underestimate the power of complete nutrition. Aloe vera, mixed with supporting vitamins and essential minerals, offers the proof of its power by its graphic ability to heal what to many has been described as beyond repair.

Thus we see some of the toughest imaginable health challenges there ever could be, wiped out easily by a natural plant.

Closing

When we look back at all we have learned regarding health, and ask ourselves again the most fundamental questions regarding the origins of illness, a new pattern emerges clearly, and it is a pattern we may apply to all pathological conditions, even new and unknown ones, when we are at a loss as to how to proceed. The most fundamental tactic of all, which underlies all methods described in this book, is simply this: restore the normal functioning of the cells. When we eat incorrectly or contaminate ourselves, we ruin cell function.

The essence of health, therefore, lies in the intake of proteins, carbs, and fats, taken in the right form as needed, with the right balance of enzymes, vitamins and minerals, in a water rich, oxygen rich environment.

Science has shown and known for decades that cells removed from the body can live forever if two vital functions are performed: one, that they are given proper nutrients and two, that their wastes are removed. You have learned how to do both in reading this book. Who knows how long you can live if you act on all you have learned?

Undoubtedly, when confronted with all of this superb research, one may ask, where have the government agencies been? Guess they somehow just missed that all of this was going on. Surely it has nothing whatsoever to do with the million dollar campaign contributions the drug companies make to politicians. We may be equally sure that even though less than 1 cent of every dollar received by the pleading government health agencies goes to any real research on disease, that all of that money is going to a worthy cause. After all, what is business without blindingly glossy advertisements for drug research? Should we not expect great results from those whose idea of research is chopping up dead animals and making guesses about what happens in life, or from those who always seem to want to study the effect of one little thing even when life is always about many little things? For consolation, we may confidently expect that at the next fundraiser, all the toothpicks will surely have rather fancy decorations, and complimentary bottles of Lorenzo's oil dressings...

The arrogance of some who endorse drugs to solve health problems can be stunning. They use hyperexpensive tools to add a hydrogen, carbon or other atom in a place nature had chosen not to, and assume their choice makes them superior. But again, think of the theory of music.

Each musician in an orchestra cannot choose his own frequency of the note A, or disharmony will result. All must tune to the same note frequency. And once one note is set, the other frequencies must all follow in a mathematically precise arrangement, else the result is noise, not music.

But all chemical compounds have frequencies, too. Perhaps man might do well to consider that nature was not incapable of making the freakish compounds whipped up by the pharmaceutical companies, but rather she chose not to, working with a sense of music lacking in the drug loving mind...

This small little book, when one takes into account the ridiculously overpriced US health care system, contains within it information worth hundreds of thousands of dollars to those who opt for a drug approach to disease. Countless problems which have led to deaths numbering at least into the hundreds of thousands, can be wiped out by a few simple adjustments.

Rest assured, if you think some scientists are angry, do not let them put you in contact with those who have lost loved ones to cancer. Be assured they are not quite as mellow as the scientists ....

It is to be hoped that every responsible citizen, upon learning of this blatant collusion among the media, government and business, might at last fulfill a public duty, and the populace at large may consider opening up enough to ask-if we see this kind of corruption in health, what kinds of car engines have been suppressed, what methods of free electricity, housing, and agriculture? What other kinds of dreams have we lost? If they are willing to protect disease for profit while generating a ghastly death toll, what else might they protect for profit? Illegal drugs? Organized crime? Global wars and terrorists for the enrichment of banks and defense contractors? Before you answer, ask yourself how well the information networks you rely on have informed you about how to stay healthy.

Stay tuned ...For if this is the tip of the iceberg, what is this titanic civilization destined for? Put another way, will we now be men, standing independently, solid and strong, or shall we remain the hollow men, the stuffed men, leaning together, headpieces filled with straw?

If the frequency work of Sharry Edwards illustrates anything, it illustrates that everything counts. Every lie we tell others affects the waveforms in our brains, and thus indelibly etches itself into our being. Every positive act rebuilds us. We do not need to wait for any cosmic justice to right that which we perceive as wrong-incorrect beliefs create their own prisons every day, every where, with every one. Correct beliefs enable our freedom the same way.

We also learn that intention is not really enough; it must be coupled with knowledge of nature's patterns, their elegance and purpose. Many will find that these methods will work for them even if they do not believe in them at all. Others with a fierce desire to heal may fail without their assistance.

Further, if we do not understand the origin of our problems, then when we use these methods and heal, we may repeat the same actions that got us sick to begin with, and start an unending cycle.

Yet we may also choose to gain natural insights and practice positive intention, and every moment, we can escape another prison, if we dare.

Thus we bring our adventure to a close. Though if you read all the references contained in this book you may find experts clashing on specific points, this book articulates where the evidence leans strongest in each instance. This may change over time, as new growth is inevitable.

You have been presented with an abundant cornucopia of natural healing self empowerment methods. The reason for this is that individuals tend to have certain preferences of their own, and one path may call out to them more than another, and each should follow their bliss. Those who follow a path they like are much more likely to follow the rules of that approach, and once again, each method does have its rules, with success determined by the extent those rules are obeyed. Further, these methods have maximum effect when parts are used wisely in combination. It is to be hoped that the larger pattern behind all these methods has been suggested to you—*they are all connected.*

To create music in our bodies, we must bring the ordered frequencies of raw nature inside us. The road to hell is paved with good intentions. The road to health is paved with good ingestions.

We exist at a most critical juncture in history, where awesome new powers and technologies lie at our fingertips, flowing amongst a populace that seems dimly aware of their existence and possibilities. Some believe very firmly that the logical conclusion of these innovative skills is paradise on earth, and as this research clearly shows, man can realize virtually any dream with enough focused effort.

We bring into reality the vision we most fully believe in.

The question now confronts you:

What do *you* believe in?

Thank you for considering the ideas of natural healing self empowerment. Please direct any questions or comments to: balancethriver@go.com

Let the adventure continue!

General Attack Plan
(To Be Used Against Any Disease When No Specific Strategy Is Ready)

Water: half as many ounces as pounds lean body weight/day (Oxywater or equivalent is ideal, but clean as you can get)
No dehydrators: coffee, typical tea (including iced), alcohol, or soft drinks
No drugs or cigarettes
Food mostly raw, enzymes used with all cooked/processed foods
Minimal refined sugars: no more than 30 grams at any one sitting, take sugars with enzymes and minerals
No freakish sugar substitutes (aspartame, splenda, etc), but natural ones (sugar alcohols) are good (xylitol, mannitol, etc)
Oxygen: take equivalent of 25 drops food grade peroxide at least half hour after last meal before going to bed (more during the day if possible)
1 gram protein/ 1 pound lean body weight /day with enzymes or less as indicated
Carbs as needed from raw foods
Fats like dairy cream, tropical oils like coconut, flax or borage
Rockland colloidal minerals or equivalent
Vitamins from raw foods
Super Papaya Enzyme Plus or equivalent enzymes when not consuming raw foods, 3 with meals, 3 between meals if overweight or needing extra detox

If skin is toxic:
Work separately with 3% food grade peroxide in a spray bottle, liquid chlorophyll, coconut oil, vinegar and/or aloe vera (or Totaloe!)

If pathogens abound:
Rockland Tox-Away, Garlic, and/or Zap 3 times a day for 2 weeks, cutting back as desired afterwards, to once a day until major symptoms gone or zapping no longer leaves you tired

If bowel movements are not proportionate to meals:
Salt water flush each morning for 40 days or until on track, break for one month, or
Rockland colon cleanse 1 month or
Super Colon Cleanse 1 month

Wait 3 days to regain strength after stopping salt water flush/bowel cleanse, then:
Liver cleanse

If in pain, enhance circulation:
Use Cardio EZ from Rockland, or
Experiment with garlic and cayenne

Next:

If toxic with heavy metals (many metal tooth fillings)
Choose to do hair analysis/urinalysis with moonlight health or Dr. Wallach if you want actual test results…
1 30 day round of chelation from moonlight health or Cardio EZ or equivalent
Liver support herbs

Wait two weeks to regain strength, then:
Master Cleanser 10-40 days

Next 2 weeks:

2 part Regeneration drinks as desired each day:

Regeneration Drinks:
Part 1)In a coffee mug or equivalent container:
1 scoop portion of Rockland whey protein or equivalent
(figure protein grams needed as *supplements*, then divide by number of drinks you plan to take each day, and have your portion: if you need 100 supplementary grams, and plan 3 drinks a day, take about 33 grams at each of 3 daily drinks)
Half and half cream to raise volume in cup about a centimeter—let your body decide the best amount
(Raw milk could replace the preceding combo)
Consume this with:
3 garlic oil triple strength capsules or equivalent
3 spirulina tablets, 3 chlorella tablets
2 enzyme supplement tablet/capsule
Next, in same cup (after emptied), mix
Part 2)1/3 of your daily dose Rockland Liquid Life Complete or equivalent
(your daily dose: 1 ounce /100 pounds lean weight /day)
100% natural fruit juice of your choice, raw preferred but not necessary
Consume this with:
3 garlic oil triple strength capsules or equivalent
1 enzyme supplement tablets/capsules

Regeneration Supplements
Rockland Cal/Mag/Potass/Boron (or equivalent) doses on the bottles or more as desired

Ease back on garlic when health appears flawless; find your own dose

Try to sleep with your body aligned north/south. Remember pets carry pathogens! If you have pets, clean them up (Dr. Wallach and Amazon herbs offer pet care products)! Read Dr. Clark's *Cure for all Diseases* for more, and read it if severely ill.

If not completely cured, go back to the top and go around again until you are. Be aware that some problems do have exotic origins: bad underground water, radiation, electromagnetic fields, toxic buildings, and others—use your diagnostic tools to pinpoint hidden origins!

About the Author
TK

I got my first library card at age 2, and have been intensely researching ever since. I have lifted weights since puberty, practiced martial art, been an ovo lacto vegetarian more than half my life, and overall the healthiest individual I know. I have never abused a drug, smoked, consumed alcohol or even one soft drink.

I am first a writer, but have been an artist, musician, mathematician, scientist, inventor, and researcher.

Several years ago, I participated in a project which resulted in the offering of a new theory of the structure of that atom. That theory can be seen online at polytope.www1.50megs.com. I tried to interest the media in listening to the theory, but they one and all refused to listen, stating that any such information could not be reviewed by mere editors, but only specialists, despite being told that the theory requires only basic math and geometry skills and public record science knowledge to understand. I discussed the theory online with scientists from over 30 countries around the world, and was surprised that 95% were supportive. But the discussions came to an end when my internet presence was sabotaged in various ways. It was strange how the fiction in the book I published, *Death of the Innovator*, had become my reality. To this day, I stand by the theory, simply because it is more accurate than the current one. To this day, the theory is ignored.

Later I began researching global corruption, eventually leading to the discovery of the book *Suppressed Inventions and Other Discoveries* by Jonathan Eisen. The health ideas presented in the book I have found accurate as far as they go, and this book represents a deeper refinement of years of research and experimentation begun from that start off point.

I do believe in the possibility of paradise on earth. Most of the tools to build such a paradise are already with us, but few are aware of them and fewer still use them.

When I think of the gift of intelligence, I aspire to live with a mankind that is worthy of that gift. Perhaps embracing the principles in this book can be a step in that direction.

I hope so.